Hope, Faith & Courage

Stories from the Fellowship of Cocaine Anonymous

Twelve Steps and Twelve Traditions
reprinted with adaptation by permission
of A.A. World Services, Inc.

Cocaine Anonymous World Services, Inc.
3740 Overland Ave. Suite C, Los Angeles, CA 90034-6337

Printed in the United States of America.

9
Library of Congress Cataloging-in-Publication Data

Hope, Faith, and Courage. *Stories from the fellowship of Cocaine Anonymous*

1. Cocaine Anonymous   2. Cocaine addicts
3. Recovery   4. Addiction

Library of Congress Catalog No. 93-74413

ISBN 0-9638193-0-5 (*Hardcover*)
ISBN 0-9638193-1-3 (*Softcover*)
ISBN 0-9638193-2-1 (*H&I edition*)

C.A. Conference-approved literature

HOPE, FAITH & COURAGE

Stories from the Fellowship of Cocaine Anonymous

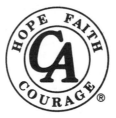

WORLD SERVICE CONFERENCE APPROVED
COCAINE ANONYMOUS WORLD SERVICES, INC.
LOS ANGELES, CALIFORNIA
1993

To the addict who still suffers...

This book, Hope, Faith, and Courage — *Stories from the Fellowship of Cocaine Anonymous*, is offered as our Fellowship's collective experience, as well as our hope that you find your own recovery. It is with heartfelt gratitude that we give this book to each of you with a resounding:

"It does work.
Keep coming back.
We're here and we're free."

Cocaine Anonymous

PREFACE

In November of 1982, several recovering addicts met and established the first Cocaine Anonymous (C.A.) group. As of 1993, our Fellowship has grown to approximately 1900 groups worldwide.

In order to make the message of hope, faith, and courage that is the spiritual center of Cocaine Anonymous more widely available, we have compiled this collection of stories recounting C.A. members' personal experiences of recovery from addiction.

For more information about Cocaine Anonymous, contact:

Cocaine Anonymous World Service Office, Inc.
P.O. Box 492000
Los Angeles, California 90049-8000

TABLE OF CONTENTS

TO THE NEWCOMER

WHO IS A COCAINE ADDICT? Some of us can answer without hesitation, "I am!" Others aren't so sure. Cocaine Anonymous believes that no one can decide for another whether he or she is addicted. One thing is sure, though: every single one of us has *denied* being an addict. For months, for years, we who now freely admit that we are cocaine addicts thought that we could control cocaine when in fact it was controlling us.

"I only use on weekends," or
"It hardly ever interferes with work," or
"I can quit, it's only psychologically addicting, right?" or
"I only snort, I don't base or shoot," or
"It's this relationship that's messing me up."

Many of us are still perplexed to realize how long we went on, never getting the same high we got in the beginning. Yet still insisting and believing — so distorted was our reality — that we were getting from cocaine what actually always eluded us.

We went to any lengths to get away from being ourselves. The lines got fatter, the grams went faster, the week's stash was all used up today. We found ourselves scraping envelopes and baggies with razor blades, scratching the last flakes from the corners of brown bottles, snorting or smoking any white speck from the floor when we ran out. We, who prided ourselves on our fine-tuned state of mind! Nothing mattered more to us than the straw, the pipe, the needle. Even if it made us feel miserable, we had to have it.

Some of us mixed cocaine with alcohol or pills, and found temporary relief in the change, but in the end, it only added to our problems. We tried quitting by ourselves, finally, and sometimes managed to do so for periods of time. After a month, we imagined we were in control. We thought our system was cleaned out and we could get the old high again, using half as much. This time, we'd be careful not to go overboard. But we only found ourselves back where we were before, and worse.

We never left the house without using first. We didn't make love without using. We didn't talk on the phone without coke. We didn't fall asleep; sometimes it seemed we couldn't even breathe without cocaine. We tried changing jobs, apartments, cities, lovers — believing that our lives were being screwed up by circumstances, places, people. Perhaps we even saw a cocaine friend die of respiratory arrest and *still* we went on using! But eventually we had to face facts. We had to admit that cocaine was a serious problem in our lives, that we were addicts.

WHAT BROUGHT US TO C.A.? Some of us hit a physical bottom. It may have been anything from a nosebleed which frightened us, to sexual impotence, to loss of sensation in or temporary paralysis of a limb, to a loss of consciousness and a trip to an emergency room, to a cocaine-induced stroke that left us disabled. Maybe it was finally our gaunt reflection in the mirror.

Others of us hit an emotional or spiritual bottom. The good times were gone, the coke life was over. No matter how much we used, we never again achieved elation, only a temporary release from the depression of coming down, and often, not even that. We suffered violent mood swings. Perhaps we awoke to our predicament after threatening or actually harming a loved one, desperately demanding imagined hidden money. We were overcome by feelings of alienation from friends, loved ones, parents, children, society, from the sky, from everything wholesome. Even the dealer we thought was our friend turned into a stranger when we went to him without money. Perhaps we awoke in dread of the isolation we had created for ourselves; using alone, suffocated by our self-centered fear and our paranoia. We were spiritually and emotionally deadened. Perhaps we thought of suicide, or tried it.

Still others of us reached a different sort of bottom when our spending and lying cost us our jobs, credit, and possessions. Some of us reached the point that we couldn't even deal; we consumed everything we touched before we could sell it. We simply could no longer afford to use. Sometimes the law intervened.

Most of us were brought down by a medley of financial, physical, social, and spiritual problems.

When we found Cocaine Anonymous, we learned that cocaine addiction is a progressive disease, chronic and potentially fatal. It fit our own experience when we heard that, contrary to popular myths about cocaine, it is possibly the most addictive substance known to man. We were relieved to be told that addiction is not simply a moral problem, that it is a true disease over which the will alone is usually powerless. All the same, each of us must take responsibility for our own recovery. There is no secret, no magic. We each have to quit and stay sober; but we don't have to do it alone!

WHAT IS COCAINE ANONYMOUS? We are a Fellowship of cocaine addicts who meet together to share our experience, strength, and hope for the purpose of staying sober and helping others achieve the same freedom. Everything heard at our meetings is to be treated as confidential. There are no dues or fees of any kind. To be a member, you only have to want to quit, and show up. We also exchange phone numbers, and give and seek support from one another between meetings.

We are all on equal footing here. There are no professional therapists offering treatment, and no one "runs" the group. Everyone in these rooms is here because he or she has a desire to stop using cocaine. We are men and women of all ages, races, and social backgrounds, with a common bond of affliction. Our Program, called the Twelve Steps of recovery, is gratefully borrowed from Alcoholics Anonymous, whose more than 50 years of experience with alcoholism teaches us that the best human help an addict can receive is from another addict. Some of us may first come to C.A. while in a treatment program or seeking individual psychotherapy. We say, "Fine, do whatever works for you." We don't pretend to have all the answers, but experience has taught us that a recovering addict will almost certainly relapse without the ongoing support of fellow addicts.

We welcome newcomers to C.A. with more genuine warmth and acceptance in our hearts than you can probably now imagine — for you are the life blood of our Program. In great part, it is by carrying the message of recovery to others like ourselves that we keep our own sobriety. We are all helping ourselves by helping each other.

WHAT IS THE FIRST THING? To the newcomer who wonders what is the first thing he or she must do to achieve sobriety, we say that you have already done the first thing: you have admitted to yourself, and now to others, that you need help by the very act of coming to a meeting or seeking information about the C.A. program.

You are also, at this very moment, doing the next thing to stay straight: you are not taking the next hit. Ours is a one-day-at-a-time program. We suggest that you should not dwell on wanting to stay sober for the rest of your life, or for a year, or even for a week. Once you have decided you want to quit, let tomorrow take care of itself. Just for today, you don't have to use. But sometimes it is too much for us to project even one whole day drug-free. That's okay. Just for the next ten minutes, you don't have to use. It's okay to want it, but you don't have to use it, just for ten minutes. After ten minutes, see where you are. You can repeat this simple process as often as necessary, using whatever span of time feels comfortable. *Just for today, you don't have to use!*

In the C.A. Fellowship, you are among recovering cocaine abusers who are living without drugs. Make use of us! Take phone numbers. Between meetings, you may not be able to avoid contact with drugs and druggies. Some of us had no sober friends at all when we first came in. You have sober friends now! When you begin to feel squirrelly, don't wait. Give one of us a call; and don't be surprised if one of us calls you when we need help!

It may surprise you that we discourage the use of *any* mind-altering substances, including alcohol and marijuana. It is the common experience of addicts in this and other programs that *any* drug use leads to relapse or substitute addiction. If you're addicted to another substance, you'd better take care of it. If you're not, then you don't need it, so why mess with it? We urge you to heed this sound advice drawn from the bitter experience of other addicts. Is it likely you're different?

We thought we were happiest with our cocaine, but we were not. In C.A., we learn to live a new way of life. We say that it is a spiritual but not a religious program — our spiritual values are accessible to the atheist as well as to the devout theist.

We who are grateful recovering cocaine addicts ask you to listen closely to our stories. That is the main thing — listen! We know where you're coming from, because we've been there ourselves. Yet we are now living drug-free, and not only that, but living happily; many of us, happier than we have ever been before. Few of us would trade all our years of addiction for the last six months or year of living the C.A. program of sobriety.

No one says that it is easy to arrest addiction. We had to give up old ways of thinking and behaving. We had to be *willing to change*. But we *are* doing it, gratefully, one day at a time.

We use the Twelve Steps[1] of recovery because it has already been proven that the Twelve Step recovery program works.

1. We admitted we were powerless over cocaine and all other mind-altering substances — that our lives had become unmanageable.

2. Came to believe that a Power greater than ourselves could restore us to sanity.

3. Made a decision to turn our will and our lives over to the care of God *as we understood Him*.

4. Made a searching and fearless moral inventory of ourselves.

5. Admitted to God, to ourselves, and to another human being the exact nature of our wrongs.

6. Were entirely ready to have God remove all these defects of character.

7. Humbly asked Him to remove our shortcomings.

8. Made a list of all persons we had harmed, and became willing to make amends to them all.

9. Made direct amends to such people wherever possible, except when to do so would injure them or others.

10. Continued to take personal inventory and when we were wrong promptly admitted it.

11. Sought through prayer and meditation to improve our conscious contact with God *as we understood Him*, praying only for knowledge of His will for us and the power to carry that out.

12. Having had a spiritual awakening as the result of these steps, we tried to carry this message to addicts, and to practice these principles in all our affairs.

There is a solution; we *can* recover from addiction. One day at a time, it is possible to live a life filled with hope, faith, and courage.

---

[1]Reprinted and adapted with permission of A.A. World Services, Inc. The Twelve Steps of Alcoholics Anonymous: 1. We admitted we were powerless over alcohol—that our lives had become unmanageable. 2. Came to believe that a Power greater than ourselves could restore us to sanity. 3. Made a decision to turn our will and our lives over to the care of God *as we understood Him*. 4. Made a searching and fearless moral inventory of ourselves. 5. Admitted to God, to ourselves, and to another human being the exact nature of our wrongs. 6. Were entirely ready to have God remove all these defects of character. 7. Humbly asked Him to remove our shortcomings. 8. Made a list of all persons we had harmed, and became willing to make amends to them all. 9. Made direct amends to such people wherever possible, except when to do so would injure them or others. 10. Continued to take personal inventory and when we were wrong promptly admitted it. 11. Sought through prayer and meditation to improve our conscious contact with God *as we understood Him*, praying only for knowledge of His will for us and the power to carry that out. 12. Having had a spiritual awakening as the result of these steps, we tried to carry this message to alcoholics, and to practice these principles in all our affairs.

The Twelve Steps and Twelve Traditions are reprinted with permission of Alcoholics Anonymous World Services, Inc. Permission to reprint and adapt the Twelve Steps and Twelve Traditions does not mean that A.A. is affiliated with this program. A.A. is a program of recovery from alcoholism. Use of the Steps and Traditions in connection with programs and activities which are patterned after A.A., but which address other problems, does not imply otherwise.

OUR HOPE, FAITH, AND COURAGE

The early days of Cocaine Anonymous as experienced by two of its members.

WHEN WE WERE asked to write the history of Cocaine Anonymous we were more than pleased, as this was a subject near and dear to us. It is a history that, as a result of timing, good fortune, and grace, we were able to experience first hand. We've had the opportunity to watch an international Fellowship grow up around us with a spirit and enthusiasm that was unfathomable to us some ten years ago[2].

We were also asked, when writing this story, in the spirit of anonymity, to exclude all names of the players involved; thus placing the focus of this recollection, as well as of this book, on the message rather than on the messengers. The fact of the matter is, that we are all somehow profoundly connected in the pursuit of physical, emotional, and spiritual sobriety. As you read the pages of this book, and hopefully relate and find strength from our experience, you will know in your heart that you, too, have become a part of the history of Cocaine Anonymous.

For the sake of clarity, I would like to explain that there are two of us writing this history. I will refer to us in this story as my partner and I; however, we are much more than that, for we are friends. We had the opportunity a few years ago to conduct a History of C.A. workshop at the World Service Convention in Arizona. We both came to Arizona armed with boxes filled with meeting directories, flyers, tickets, newspaper and magazine clippings, letters, T-shirts, and minutes of business meetings dating back to the beginning of this Fellowship. We sat cross-legged in that elegant hotel

---

[2] The first meeting of Cocaine Anonymous was held in November 1982.

room, two recovering drug addicts, sorting through papers, swapping stories, laughing and crying about so many events that had chiseled out the course of our lives.

In November, 1982, I had been clean and sober for about five months. Prior to that, I had slipped in and out of sobriety in Alcoholics Anonymous for just over a year. I had been a fan in a fellowship where only players grew and thrived. The concept of "being willing to go to any length" was only just then beginning to mean something to me.

One November afternoon, I received a call from a person who had been instrumental in my initial sobriety. This individual, sober for many years already, was calling to inform me of an A.A. meeting at the Motion Picture and Television Fund, in Hollywood, California, that was to take place on the following Tuesday. The topic was to be drugs, especially cocaine. Apparently, the Motion Picture and Television Fund had been flooded with calls from members and others, seeking help for cocaine addiction. Despite the fact that the community at large still considered cocaine to be a nonaddictive drug, there seemed to be an epidemic of nonaddicted, addicted people. I was very excited at the prospect of this meeting. I had been addicted to cocaine, alcohol, pills, psychedelics, opiates, and anything else I could get my hands on. The thought of a forum in which men and women could discuss the solutions of the Twelve Steps and Twelve Traditions in relation to their common experience of bondage to cocaine was most intriguing to me.

The meeting began as does any meeting in Southern California, with the reading of "Chapter Five," from the Big Book of Alcoholics Anonymous[3]. It quickly took on

---

[3] At the sixth C.A. World Service Conference, held in 1989, a motion was passed to approve the advisory opinion, "The books *Alcoholics Anonymous* and *Twelve Steps and Twelve Traditions* of Alcoholics Anonymous are two of our most valuable tools of recovery and as such, it is the opinion of Cocaine Anonymous that meetings should be allowed to have these books available to support members in their recovery."

an electrifying new dimension. Words like basing, snorting, shooting, copping, scoring, dealing, paranoia, and depression went flying around the room with heads nodding and bursts of laughter — our way of expressing the fact that we relate. One member shared about snorting lint from a shag carpet while searching for a rock. Another talked of the desperate feelings of seeing the light come through the corners of the sheets covering the windows, hearing the deafening sound of the morning birds, and of wanting to take his .45 magnum and "waste" those birds; but being afraid to go outside the house because "they" might be out there.

Just prior to the close of this meeting, it was suggested that we take a group conscience to turn this Alcoholics Anonymous meeting into a completely new Twelve Step program, and call it Cocaine Anonymous. This motion, which sounded like a wonderful idea to me, was quickly voted down. I remember being upset at the time, only to realize later that my thinking had been incorrect; turning an A.A. meeting into a C.A. meeting would have completely disregarded the Twelve Traditions. We would have been trying to turn an apple into an orange. Although they have much in common, they are simply different fruits.

Directly after the meeting that evening, it occurred to a few of us that there was plenty of room and time for both apples and oranges. This was a Tuesday night. We were told by our friend at the Motion Picture and Television Fund that if we returned on Thursday night, there would be a room for us.

Two days later we returned with great anticipation. Approximately twenty members; men and women, newcomers and old-timers from all walks of life, sat in silence at the sound of knuckles hitting the top of a wooden table. A voice I will never forget said, "Welcome to the first Cocaine Anonymous meeting. My name is _____, and I'm an addict and an alcoholic. Cocaine Anonymous is a fellowship of men and women who share their experience, strength, and hope with each other that they may solve their common problem and help others recover from their addiction." At that moment, you could have heard a pin drop. There was electricity in that room. I believe that as a group, we intuitively knew that something very important had happened, an event that would not just affect our lives, but the lives of countless others for years to come.

At about the same period of time, a hospital in Los Angeles had begun a closed, patient-only meeting, established for addicts whose primary drug was cocaine. Shortly after the inception of Cocaine Anonymous, this hospital meeting opened its doors to all addicts. It became one of the original six Cocaine Anonymous meetings, meetings which seemed to pop up overnight. These became six places a week for cocaine addicts to experience recovery in a safe, supportive environment, where all that was asked of them was to have a desire to be free from their addiction, and to help other addicts achieve the same freedom.

With the existence of these six meetings came the beginning of C.A.'s first attempt to establish a service organization. What this boiled down to was this: each meeting had its secretary represent it at the first service meeting. Given the fact that there were so few of us in attendance, we all miraculously ended up on the Board of Directors. That evening, I made the acquaintance of two other members who were, like myself, driven for some inexplicable reason to devote their next few years to the development and growth of Cocaine Anonymous. Although we were strangers at first and agreed on very little, we quickly developed a strong bond, friendship, and singleness of purpose. Looking back now, I know that we were not being noble; we were simply saving our lives, though none of us realized anything that uncomplicated then.

All three of us, with less than a year of sobriety, along with others, would meet at my house a couple of times a week to discuss, argue, and finally agree on subjects ranging from public information, to literature, to phone lines, to chips, to what to order for dinner that evening. We were starting from scratch, with nothing to lose but our slavery to drugs.

Our first chairperson excelled in his ability to organize. My strong point, as vice-chair, was my ability to motivate and organize others. My partner, whom I referred to before, was a serious stickler for details. He became the office manager; although, at the time, we didn't actually have an office. We did, however, have a phone and an answering machine. This was our first method used to reach out and be available to addicts who were looking for a meeting, and members around the country who wanted to start meetings in their area.

If you happened to have called in that first year, you would have received a prompt call back from my partner, our office manager. However, chances are, in the first few months of his job, there would have been two people grinding their teeth during that conversation. Unbeknownst to us, my partner was still using periodically, during which time he spoke at length, might I add, and Twelfth Stepped many people, who years later are still active members.

The phone also became an embarrassment and a lesson to us when we realized that we were compromising the Traditions of C.A.[4] The phone lines were paid for, and located in, a local drug recovery hospital. We justified this at first, because we were virtually broke, and the phone lines enabled us to reach out. As we began to grow spiritually in our own sobriety, and began to accept guidance from supportive members of Alcoholics Anonymous and Narcotics Anony-

---

[4] See Appendix I for the Twelve Traditions of Cocaine Anonymous.

mous[5], it became all too clear that without our adherence to, and respect for, the Twelve Traditions, we risked the integrity and the very existence of Cocaine Anonymous. We learned we had to be self-supporting through our own contributions, and had to have faith that we would grow accordingly.

There was controversy in those early days that came from those who believed we were unnecessary, that we existed as an "emergency room clearing house" to other fellowships, or that we simply wouldn't survive as a fellowship. We, on the other hand, had read a pamphlet written by the founder of A.A. called *Problems Other Than Alcohol*, which encouraged us to move forward on our quest and not become part of the controversy. As it turned out, the controversy shortly dissolved into open arms and cooperation from all involved.

It was our hope that the C.A. chips would be a unifying factor in our young Fellowship — something solid to touch, to carry with us, a reminder of our commitment. At that time, we had a hard, white, square chip with letters and numbers. These unfortunately would wear off before you could even get to the next meeting, not to mention that relapsers would use the chips to chop cocaine. In moving to a rounded, more flexible chip, I was asked to come up with three words that would epitomize the spirit of Cocaine Anonymous. Originally, these words were "Hope, Faith, and Willingness." Unfortunately, we had to discard the word "Willingness" because it had too many letters. That evening, I sat at home watching a television documentary on President Kennedy. He spoke eloquently on the necessity of having "courage" in our lives. It occurred to me that when many of us walk through the doors of Cocaine Anonymous for the first time,

---

[5] The Fellowship of Cocaine Anonymous is grateful to individual members of Alcoholics Anonymous (A.A.) and Narcotics Anonymous (N.A.) for their cooperation in our beginning and subsequent survival; however, these references are not meant to imply affiliation.

we do so without hope, without faith, but with an ounce of *courage*. We listen to the stories and experiences of others and develop *hope*. As a result of coming back, and coming back, and coming back and working the Twelve Steps, we acquire an abundance of *faith*. Thus were born the guiding principles *Hope*, *Faith*, and *Courage*.

One evening, sitting in an all-night diner with a good friend (whom my partner ironically Twelfth Stepped, while working the phones "under the influence"), trying to write a suggested standardized meeting format, I found myself deep in discussion about what I believed to be our most pressing obstacle. As women and men came into C.A. they were able, through our fellowship and example, and guidance from the Steps, to give up the use of cocaine, and begin a new life. Unfortunately, many members refused to stop using other substances, explaining that they weren't alcoholics, that pot was a natural herb, or that they really needed those pills to relax or sleep in such a stressful period as early recovery, etc., etc. These members, who usually relapsed on cocaine or began abusing their new drug of choice, often punctuated their case with the challenge, "Anyway, where does it mention anything other than cocaine?" That evening, over a plate of greasy bacon and eggs we rewrote the First Step, simply adding after the word cocaine: "and all other mind-altering substances." — five little words that almost overnight put to rest this dangerous, life-threatening debate — five little words that told the demons in my head to surrender.

Within a year, the Fellowship had grown to 30 meetings. The days of a handful of us representing the group conscience were over. It was fun while it lasted. But frankly, we were grateful to share the responsibility. For some reason (which eludes me now), the 30 representatives of these 30 meetings decided that we could get more work done if we went on a group service retreat. I still laugh when I think of the chaos and drama that went on between us all; some in our second year, most in their first year, many in their first few months.

The weekend retreat took place at a monastery in the high desert. Respecting the monks' traditions, we ate breakfast in silence. But we never stopped bickering the rest of the day. Like so many other challenges we were meeting in our new clean and sober lives, by the end of this weekend we had developed a sense of community and a feeling of unity.

The weekend ended with a C.A. meeting in the monks' cemetery at the close of a clear, beautiful day. We each took our turn, sharing our gratitude and love, as the sun began to set and a cold wind blew across the desert floor. Suddenly, interrupting a particularly heartfelt share, one of the representatives (with three months off freebase) reached into his pocket and cried out, "Oh no!" He pulled out a rather large plastic bag filled with cocaine. Thirty hearts began to race. Thirty minds began to run. As a group, we simply froze. The thought of the entire service structure of C.A. being wiped out in an afternoon was too absurd. Someone nervously suggested we take a group conscience. Another member jokingly proposed we sell the blow and donate the profits. Before this event got too out of hand, before the sun set altogether beyond the horizon, with the last bits of light shooting across the desert, a large gust of wind arose. This wise newcomer opened the bag, grabbed the bottom, and began to wave it in the air. In a moment, a cloud of white powder went floating away into the twilight. We sat there as a group in silence, as if we were saying goodbye to an old friend. We were in awe at the knowledge that together, with the help of a Higher Power, we could do what individually had always eluded us. We held hands, said the Serenity Prayer, and went home.

During the next two and one-half years, C.A. grew at a remarkable rate. As the result of articles about "the cocaine epidemic and recovery" that mentioned Cocaine Anonymous in the *Los Angeles Times*, *People*, *Time*, and *Newsweek*, inquiries about the Program began to flow in. We were overwhelmed by this response. It became apparent to us, especially my partner, that the time for a world service organization had arrived. Our amazing growth in California was paralleled by C.A. fellowships cropping up in several cities throughout the United States.

Within this time period, we received an envelope from the Chicago Fellowship that contained a pamphlet they had written and were offering for our consideration, in hopes it would become C.A.'s first piece of literature. We, in the California contingency, had been working very hard on a piece already. But between us, we couldn't agree on a single page. With tremendous skepticism, we sat and read aloud this bold offering from this far away place. It was perfect. With mouths hanging open and tears in our eyes, we knew that these words said exactly what needed to be said. It was entitled *To the Newcomer* and includes what is now referred to as "Who Is a Cocaine Addict," which is read aloud at many meetings throughout the world.

On May 3, 1985, hundreds of recovering addicts converged on a beachfront hotel in Santa Barbara, California, to attend the first annual World Service Convention. It was called the Seaside Unity and Acceptance Convention, but was much, much, more than that. Voices from the phone and names from letters were taking form. Faces of old friends we had not as yet met appeared there before us. From coast-to-coast we came — excited, curious and filled with an energy that was to become our trademark.

In a crowded room on a Saturday morning, the diligent chairperson of World Services cautiously called to order the first national business meeting. After a passionate exchange of ideas, which set the format for future conferences, the meeting came to a close with a remarkable feeling of optimism.

That night we gathered together in the hotel's banquet hall to feast and celebrate our new Fellowship. Men and women who had only recently graced bathrooms, prisons, mental wards, and treatment centers were now seated in this balloon-filled majestic room, shoulder-to-shoulder, looking and feeling alive and well. The speaker was inspiring to our already high-spirited group. Banquet food even seemed to taste good that night. The first chairperson, and my partner and I were recognized that evening as C.A.'s first Trustees. This recognition somehow represented to us, and to those present, the spiritual connection and acceptance of what was, and what could be in the future. The highlight of the evening was the state-by-state countdown. One-by-one, each participating state was announced. Its representatives rose to the cheers and applause that grew to a fevered pitch, as voices cried out: "Alaska, Arizona, California, Connecticut, District of Columbia, Georgia, Hawaii, Illinois, Nevada, New Jersey, New York, Ohio, Tennessee, Texas, Virginia, Washington, and Wisconsin."

In the years since that convention, C.A. has spread its message and enthusiasm throughout the United States, beyond the border to Canada, and across the Atlantic Ocean to Europe.[6]

When I was newly sober it was explained to me that the Greek definition of the word "enthusiasm" is, "en," meaning 'in' or 'with,' and "theos" meaning 'God.' In other words — having God within. One day at a time, the Fellowship of Cocaine Anonymous enthusiastically carries the message of Cocaine Anonymous throughout the world to the addict who

---

[6] The Cocaine Anonymous World Service Office has received requests for Meeting Starter Kits from around the world.

has the courage to ask for help.

A while back, I had a most disturbing dream. It began like a retrospective collage, covering my clean and sober years. I dreamt of friends and lovers whose wisdom had altered my damaged way of thinking, of events like those covered in this story: the wonder of the first C.A. meeting and the excitement of the Seaside Unity and Acceptance Convention. I dreamt of working the Steps and experiencing a new sense of well-being, blended perfectly with a rebirth of my passion. I dreamt of courage, hope, and faith, of learning that "success may be getting what you want, but happiness is wanting what you get."

All at once, in a flash, I dreamt that I awoke. Still dreaming, I believed that all my clean and sober years had never happened. That I was again "coming to" that day, still caught in the horrifying grips of a progressive state of high anxiety, loneliness, despair, and addiction. My body filled with spasms, my mind with paranoia, my spirit deadened; I was pathetic. These thoughts hurled me into a state of panic.

I broke out in a sweat, my eyes flew open, and at last I was awake, for real. Still groggy and frightened, I shook as I tried to remember what was true. Slowly but surely, I took a deep breath, got into the moment and knew that everything was as it should be; I wasn't alone. I was clean and sober; I had experienced a complete psychic change; I was safe.

Suddenly, I was overcome with a clear euphoric sensation, as I intuitively understood that even if the nightmare had been true, even if I was still back in the land of hopelessness, chances are I might still find help. All at once, I had the revelation that what I would have to do is get out of bed, get dressed, find another addict with the courage to change, and tell him about my dream.

PERSONAL STORIES

Twenty-seven recovering addicts share their hope, faith, and courage.

1

TRUE FREEDOM

A prison sentence during recovery helped this man to appreciate true inner freedom — freedom from self.

I NOW REALIZE that I had the characteristics of addiction long before I crossed the thin line between being a drug abuser and an addict. It wasn't until I applied these traits to a substance called cocaine that I realized I had met my match. Of course, this wasn't until after years of trying to control my use of cocaine, because my pride and ego would not let me admit defeat to a white powdery substance. This, in addition to the fact that I was a drug hustler, kept me in denial. I was addicted to the drama of selling drugs. The false sense of winning and power that comes with selling drugs helped enable my addiction. I started out winning financially more than I lost, until I became my best customer. My addiction to the fast life, the vicious cycle of buying and selling, the false friends, the risks, and the adventure started long before I was introduced to cocaine.

I started with marijuana when I was thirteen. I tried it all, from uppers to downers, from angel dust to alcohol. It was cool with a certain clique at my high school to get high, and I was willing to go to any length to fit in.

My father was a recording engineer and he had built a soundproof studio in our basement. This led me to become a musician. There has always been a myth that a musician has to get high to get into the groove; so I used this as just another excuse to justify my getting high at such a young age. As my disease progressed, so did my desire for the immediate gratification of fast money. There was an added bit of glamour to my career. As a musician I had learned the ropes of

1

getting backstage at many of the concerts in my hometown. Therefore, not only would I get to party with lots of celebrities and musicians but I could supplement my income by dealing at the same time.

Somehow, I had always done well in school. I made the dean's list my first year in college. I decided to work a full-time job and continue my education later. I got a job at a major bank where I eventually got a position as a computer operator. I worked there for eight and one-half years. I thought that I was slick and had it all together. All of this was about to go rapidly down the drain.

Over the years, I ran into better sources for my drugs. One day I went to meet my connection who I did not know was being watched by the Drug Enforcement Administration. I'll never forget that day; it was Friday the thirteenth. I had taken the day off work. I started the day with a bowl of cereal and a hit off the cocaine pipe. I still had plenty of product and profit left from a sale I had made the night before. Being the greedy addict that I am, I wanted to make sure that I had enough for myself and enough to sell for the weekend ahead. I called and placed an order and was instructed when and where to meet my connection. When I met him, he gave me twice the amount I had ordered and said, "This way I won't have to see you for a while." That's when the D.E.A. moved in and busted me red-handed. I fought my case in court for the next two years. During this time, I lost my job at the bank. I continued to use drugs, but on a smaller scale, because my sources thought I was too big a risk to deal to.

I can vividly remember the last time I got high. By then, I was in the habit of blowing my paycheck every Friday in twenty-five-dollar increments. Each time I would tell myself that I was just going to get one package, smoke it, and stop. This particular Friday was no exception. I was at one of my favorite crack houses. When I arrived at 5:00 P.M., the guy who ran the house acted like my best friend. When all my money was gone by 3:00 A.M., he kicked me out. I was frustrated because I couldn't get that blast I was chasing. It took all I had to hold on to some sense of pride and dignity.

I felt like an empty shell of a man. My physical appearance wasn't much better. At 5'11", I weighed about 135 pounds. I had once again neglected all responsibilities to my loved ones and creditors. I didn't know how to love myself, so how could I love anyone else? My girlfriend had no understanding of the disease of addiction. She and my three-year-old daughter were forced to share the horrors of my addiction because she didn't want to give up on me.

When I left the crack house that night, I ran into a fellow addict who was looking for a sting so he could get another package. I really didn't know him well, but he reminded me of myself. We shared a common objective — one more hit. We only had about ten dollars between the two of us, but he eventually found some guys to con out of their money. We were off to the races again. We went to his house, where he said we could have some privacy. When we got there, all he had was a broken piece of a glass pipe. As I sat back and watched him put his lips around that broken pipe, I saw myself. I shook my head and said, "I can't go on living like this." However, as soon as it was my turn, I wrapped my lips around that same broken pipe. I still couldn't get the satisfaction that I was looking for. I left his house totally disgusted and depressed. My pride and ego were now thoroughly crushed.

I arrived home, and walked through the door like a wet puppy with his tail between his legs. However, this time something was different. It was almost as if my girlfriend had stopped caring. I was no longer able to manipulate her by playing on her sympathy. She simply said, "You've got to get some help or we are leaving."

The next day I called a treatment center. One of the reasons I had put it off for so long was because I was afraid my employer would fire me when he found out that I had a drug problem. I was assured that my 28-day stay would be strictly confidential. I packed my bags, and they took me in right away. When I heard the similarities in the stories of the other residents, I knew that I was where I belonged. I was relieved to find out that I was a sick person and not a bad person, that I suffered from an incurable disease that could be arrested one day at a time, as long as I stayed away from the first drink or drug.

This is where I was first introduced to Cocaine Anonymous and the Twelve Step program of recovery. I didn't have much of a problem with the first three Steps, because I had always believed and had faith in my Higher Power, which I chose to call God. My biggest problem was how long I could stay out of the driver's seat after turning my life over to God. I was in the habit of jumping back behind the wheel as soon as God put me back on my feet. Well, C.A. has a simple suggestion for this problem — one day at a time.

Meanwhile, my attorney was still stalling in court by getting a continuance every month. So I kept going to meetings, got a sponsor, did service work, and began to reap one of the greatest rewards of the Program, a sense of serenity that money can't buy. The judge sentenced me to four years in prison for possession of cocaine. However, since I had a job and a family, he gave me five days to tie up my business and turn myself in. These were the hardest five days of my sobriety. I felt like God had betrayed me until I realized that I had been bargaining with God in the back of my mind. I wanted to work toward recovery in exchange for God helping me beat my case. To make it through those five days I used the tools of the Program: the telephone, the Serenity Prayer, my sponsor, and daily meetings. I was tired of running. I had been escaping from the realities of life through the last fifteen years of my drug use. I had to cling to my faith that one day I would realize my Higher Power was allowing me to go through this experience for a reason, and that it was best for me.

Five days later, I turned myself in. From that point on, I chose to make time serve me rather than to serve time. I felt as though I had been serving time in bondage during the fifteen years I had been getting high. I refused to waste any more of my life. I had a taste of the freedom that recovery had given me in the five months prior to being sentenced. My fear of returning to the bondage of active addiction was stronger than my fear of dealing with life on life's terms. I stayed busy in prison by making meetings, reading spiritual and program literature, playing my guitar, and working out with weights. I set up a daily routine of discipline because I wanted to establish some good habits for when I returned to society. I took the time to work the Steps as rigorously as I could.

After six months in prison, I was allowed to go to a work-release camp for the next fifteen months. They didn't have a Twelve Step meeting at that facility when I arrived, so I helped to start the first meeting. I used the Serenity Prayer often to deal with the insanity I was surrounded by. Most of all, I learned the true meaning of freedom. Even though I was incarcerated I was grateful to be free from the horrors of active addiction I could remember so vividly. I could still remember the hopeless feeling of being out of control after taking that first drink or drug. After 21 months, I was released on parole.

Today, I have committed my life to service work in C.A. My life is continually getting better. I still tend to jump into the driver's seat occasionally, but when I get into enough pain and humiliation I "let go and let God." I am now happily married. I'm fulfilling some of my life's dreams and ambitions by studying music and pursuing a career in the music industry. My wife and I are in the process of relocating our family to a city in which I have always wanted to live. I owe it all to the Fellowship and Twelve Steps of C.A. for helping me to find the faith in my Higher Power and to strive for a better way of life.

2

THE FUNCTIONAL ADDICT

This addict functioned out in the world, but was dying inside until his life was turned around by Cocaine Anonymous and an understanding of the words "no matter what."

*M*Y BEST FRIEND had been knocking on the door for several minutes. Neither he nor anyone else was expected. I eased the needle out of my arm, found myself at the door and angrily yanked it open. The sight that greeted my friend was one of me naked except for a pair of bikini underwear, a sheen of sweat covering my body, my eyes crazed, and bright red blood trickling down my left arm towards my wrist. I told him not to dare ever darken my door again without calling first, and slammed the door in his face and on our relationship. Today, that relationship has been repaired and is one of the many gifts I've received from the program of Cocaine Anonymous.

I am an addict of the worst kind. When I say, "I am an addict," I mean that I deny, discount, minimize, and medicate my feelings. The exception is rage, which I have never minimized in my life. Rather, I expressed it inappropriately and in amounts disproportionate to what a situation called for. I also mean that when given a good reason to stop using cocaine, I could not, and that once I started using, I had no control over the amount I consumed.

When I say, "I am an addict of the worst kind," I mean that I am a functional addict. When I hit my bottom, I held a position at a prestigious hospital in Southern California, taught at a major university, and spent much of my time traveling around the country lecturing. I still had my home, car, and marriage. This empowered my denial. When you came to me to tell me you were worried about me because you

7

thought I was killing myself with cocaine, I could say to you, "When you have my job, teach where I teach, are as successful as I, then talk to me about my problem. Until then, just mind your own business. I can stop anytime I want to; I just don't want to right now."

I also need to say that, given my history with other drugs, alcohol, food, sugar, needles, cigarettes, incest, sexual behavior, guns, stealing, and violence, I could have ended up in the morgues of many cities, in hospitals, in prisons, or in any of a number of Twelve Step programs. But I did not. Instead, I found my way to Cocaine Anonymous. Our Preamble states that we share our experience, strength, and hope, but I have found that we share much more. Yes, we share experience, strength, and hope, but we also share our hearts, our time, our ears, our shoulders, our arms, our love, and whatever else it takes to keep ourselves and one another sober, one day at a time. I am proud to be a member of this Fellowship.

I don't pretend to understand my disease or its origins. I was born into a functional family that was very much in love with the idea of having a baby. However, the idea of having a baby and the reality of caring for one were very different. After four or five months of changing diapers and feeding me, my mother left, never to return. I do not know if this had anything to do with the way in which I used drugs and alcohol — addictively. My father remarried a wonderful woman around my third birthday. She has been my mother since then.

By the time I was three and one-half years old, my parents were in a working situation which kept them from being home during the week. Therefore, I stayed with a family of eight (six kids, a mom and a dad) during the week, and with my parents on the weekends. I was sexually, physically, and emotionally brutalized by the father and oldest teenage son of that family. I was sodomized, beaten, locked in dark closets, and threatened on an ongoing basis between the ages of three and one-half and four and one-half. I do not know if this "made" me an addict and alcoholic. Today that is not important. I do know that others have walked similar gauntlets and emerged without becoming addicts or alcoholics.

During this period of my abuse, my parents had a huge cocktail party every Saturday night. It was there that my drinking began. I was the cute little kid, in a suit and tie, who went around and drank the bottom of everyone's drinks until I passed out. The party guests thought it cute to see the little boy in his suit being a bit tipsy and then being carried to bed.

When I was four and one-half, my parents discovered that I was being abused, pulled me out of that situation, changed their jobs, and we moved away. There were no more weekly parties, and there was no more alcohol. However, sugar, food, books, daydreams, and fantasies quickly took the place of alcohol, and were used addictively. In the next eight years we moved many times. I was always the new kid, the poor kid, the fat kid, the only child, and the kid who was teased.

I felt less than, not a part of, different, and more than anything, a victim. If I learned anything from my abandonment, sexual abuse, and frequent relocations, it was how to think of myself as a victim. I hurt more than you, was lonelier than you, and carried pain that was beyond the comprehension of anyone but my dog (a dog which I was forced to give up in the midst of one of our many moves). I was awash with self-pity, a self-pity that served to isolate me and that I used to justify myriad indulgences and self-destructive behaviors.

I was also filled with self-loathing and self-hatred which grew from a fear of and an unwillingness to fight or defend myself when I was picked on as the new kid. That changed, however, the summer between seventh and eighth grades. On my twelfth birthday, my biologic mother called to say that although she had not seen me for almost twelve years, she wanted to make peace, have me meet my two half-brothers (she had remarried), and spend the summer with her and her new family. I agreed to go when school let out. The night before I was to leave, she called to say that she had changed her mind, that I could not come because I would be too difficult to explain to their neighbors. With that news, something inside of me snapped, and I lost my fear of fighting. I quickly became one of the bad boys, eager to fight, to hurt, and to engage in destructive acts. I surrounded myself with lower companions who were of the same ilk. We proceeded to fight, hurt, destroy, and get loaded.

From there, my getting loaded only progressed. I dropped out of high school during my senior year and found my way to Greenwich Village in the mid-sixties. I smoked weed and hash, took a lot of acid, and put down the junkies who stuck needles in their arms and the straights who drank martinis. Little did I know that needles and martinis would eventually work their way to the top of my list of priorities.

I returned home and went to work at a top nightclub. I was the baby there. I was taken under the waitress' wings and taught the ways of the world. This included how to drink, shoot dope, and sell dope right through the box office window. I snorted my first cocaine in the dressing rooms and light booth of this club. I spent the first of a fortune of dollars on cocaine there, as well. My very first purchase of cocaine was in an amount greater than my monthly rent.

For years I used cocaine, initially in a controlled manner, but addictively after crossing that imaginary line separating the casual user from the addict. I used it when it was fun and worked, and continued to use it long after it stopped working. My drug use led me to armed robbery which earned me a sentence of five years to life in state prison, where I was raped. It still didn't occur to me that perhaps I had a drug problem. Remember, I had expertise at being a victim and a blamer of others for my woes.

I came out of prison and went to a community college. I did well as a science major and won a full academic scholarship to a major university. While there, I stopped snorting coke and returned to shooting it. In every bathroom on the campus, I have sat in a stall, drawn toilet water into a syringe, mixed it with my coke, and jammed it into my arm. I gave up my dreams of getting into veterinary school. I did go on to earn my Master's degree and distinguish myself in my professional field.

I managed to stop shooting coke. I returned to snorting it on a constant basis, and drinking just as constantly "to take the edge off." I tried to stop, swore I'd stop, made promises to stop, but could not. I tried just saying no, and as I was saying no, my fingers would dial the dealer's or liquor store's phone number. The humiliation of bankruptcy did not help me stop. Drunk-driving arrests did not help me stop. Even when the drugs and alcohol no longer made me feel good and no longer numbed the pain, I could not stop. When I could not stop, I tried to change and limit when and how much I used; at this too, I failed completely. I felt out of control and like a failure.

Near the end of my using, the quality of my marriage had all but disappeared. We were more like good using and drinking buddies than like husband and wife. There was ample fighting and getting loaded, but no respect, communication, or tenderness. The two of us were like an island, totally isolated from those who had been our friends. They had all pulled away, either out of anger over our outrageous alcoholic behavior or because they loved us so much they could simply no longer watch us kill ourselves. I felt completely alone.

Near the end of my using, I was also exhausted both physically and emotionally. I was scared, angry, and indignant that the drugs no longer worked. I was filled with self-loathing, self-righteousness, and self-pity. Why was this happening to me, poor me? I could no longer look at myself

in the mirror because of my self-hatred. Completely demor-
alized, I knew my only answer was suicide. It would end my
misery, and certainly my wife would be better off with my
sizable insurance money than with me.

I carefully planned my suicide to look like an accident so
that the insurance benefits would be larger. On the afternoon
I intended to kill myself, I was sitting at home drinking gin,
tooting coke, and not feeling any better. The television was
on, and one of those cocaine ads that I had seen many times
before came on. This time, instead of throwing a finger at the
television, I burst into tears and called the number listed. I
stayed on the C.A. hotline for 90 minutes with the recovering
addict who answered the phone. He told me that there was a
meeting starting shortly near my house, and that I should go
to it.

I stumbled into that meeting too loaded to remember
anything. I *do* remember that after the meeting, a gentle man
sat me down over some coffee and told me three things that
stuck: 1) I never again had to feel the way I felt at that moment;
2) he and C.A. would love me until I learned to love myself;
and 3) I never had to drink or use again, one day at a time.

I spent the next couple of days on my couch, sick as a dog.
I then went to another meeting. There, the speaker drew an
analogy between this Program and the story of the great artist
Michelangelo. When asked how he had created the brilliant
sculpture of David, Michelangelo replied, "I just got a big
block of marble and chipped away everything that wasn't
David." As I sat crying like a baby, I somehow knew that this
Program would enable me to chip away everything that
wasn't me, and it is doing just that. At my third meeting, I
heard a woman speak whose story was nothing like mine, but
whose feelings had been identical. At that moment, I knew I
was home and that everything would be okay. The next day
I asked her to be my sponsor. Though she declined, she

directed me to a man who became, and remained, my sponsor for the first two and one-half years of my sobriety.

I cannot tell you why I got this Program. I know that I was willing, and that I held no illusions about the drugs working again some day. I was through; the drugs and alcohol didn't work anymore. It was this Program or suicide. When I went to meetings, I knew I was loved, cared for, and would be okay.

My wife did not get sober when I did. In fact, she continued to drink and use in increasing quantities for the first few months of my sobriety. When I'd come home from work, the house would smell like pot and there would be drugs and alcohol everywhere. But I did not drink or use. I knew in my heart that that part of my life was over. I took direction from my sponsor. I tried to be an attraction to her, rather than trying to promote the Program or get her sober. Shortly thereafter, my wife raised her hand in a meeting, identified as an alcoholic, and has been sober ever since. Today, as I write this, it is our twenty-second wedding anniversary. That we are both alive and together in a loving relationship is truly a gift of the Program.

With the guidance of a loving sponsor, I have worked the Steps of this Program. Being an atheist, I had some trouble with Steps Two and Three. However, I did my best and made the Group of Drug addicts at the meetings my GOD initially. I hit my knees twice daily simply as an exercise in humility, rather than in faith or belief. I turned my will and my life over by working Steps Four through Nine to the best of my ability. As I did, I found a faith and a belief in a Power greater than myself. Today there is a God in my life. It is not a bearded guy in the sky who punishes and rewards me, but a force in my heart which can free me and to which I pray daily. I ask for the willingness and ability to stay in touch with and radiate the dignity, grace, love, and energy which dwell within my heart.

On my Ninth Step, I found it necessary to make amends to myself before anyone else, for I had damaged myself more than anyone else. I do a daily Tenth Step mentally, and a written one twice a week. I pray on a daily basis and meditate some of the time. Finally, I do try to live and carry the message. Most importantly, I try to practice surrender, love, honesty, hope, faith, courage, responsibility, gratitude, humility, charity, tolerance, acceptance, forgiveness, and service in all my affairs. I try to bring an attitude of service to every situation I find myself in today. I do this because I find that the attitude and action of service encompasses most of the previously mentioned principles, keeps me clean and sober, in the solution, and in touch with God.

I did hit a wall in my sobriety at about ten months. Problems with work, money, my relationship, and having gotten in touch with my childhood incest seemed overwhelming. I did not want to use or drink, but found myself very suicidal. A friend made me promise that not only would I not use cocaine, but also that I wouldn't kill myself, *no matter what*. I certainly understood intellectually what the words *no matter what* meant, but I did not understand them in my heart. Then I heard a story from another friend which brought that meaning home to my heart, saved my life, and became my *no matter what* story.

This friend used cocaine the same way I did, and got sober the same way I did, in the rooms of Cocaine Anonymous. A while into his sobriety, he started dating a girl, fell in love with her, and eventually became engaged to her. One day they went skydiving together and she was killed in an accident. One day at a time, my friend did not drink or use *no matter what*. Rather, he came to the rooms of Cocaine Anonymous. And there he found a place where he could rage and cry. There he found a fellowship of men and women ready to share, not just their experience, strength, and hope, but their hearts, their time, their ears, their shoulders, their arms, their love, and whatever else it took to keep themselves, and him, sober one day at a time, *no matter what.*

Upon hearing that story, I understood *no matter what.* Today when things seem overwhelming, I simply think of my friend staying sober through his loss, and I don't drink, use, or kill myself, one day at a time, *no matter what.*

I am not alone anymore. I am a proud and grateful member of Cocaine Anonymous, and thank C.A. for giving me my life, a God, and the opportunity to give to others.

3

AMERICA BY CARS & BARS
A half-step became Twelve Steps.

S A LITTLE girl, I didn't dream of growing up to be a drug addict. I always hated drugs. I would cry and yell when my older brother and sister came home with friends and smoked pot. A few years later, when other friends were singing songs by The Partridge Family, I was singing the lyrics of the Grateful Dead. I had no way of knowing then that those songs would describe my life in years to come.

I was thirteen or so when I first drank. Right from the start, I drank to get drunk, to get out of myself, to be comfortable in a group of people. I was always scared and insecure. I found that beer changed the way I felt inside, and I liked it. I always felt different — uncool, like everyone else was cool but me.

It was cool, I thought, to shoplift; so I started doing that for attention. I always stole stuff for other people, never for myself. When I got caught, I convinced (manipulated is a better word) my mother that I was stealing as a result of my parents' divorce. I knew she felt guilty about the divorce and that this manipulation would work. It did. She cried a lot. Inside, I was laughing because I'd gotten away with it!

I started smoking pot, again to be cool and to feel a part of the group. I never dared tell anyone that I didn't know what the high should feel like. I never said, "I don't really like this stuff, do you?" I just imitated what the stoned people did. I began to ignore that voice inside me that told me right from wrong, and what I liked and didn't like. That was the little voice that let me know who I was. I silenced it with drugs until I got into the Fellowship of Cocaine Anonymous.

When I went away to college, I was scared, insecure, and still felt less than everyone else. I began to go to happy hour regularly. Before long, school took a back-burner to partying. I'd always been a good student. Now I was getting mostly incompletes. I lost all desire to go to school.

I took a summer job at a resort hotel. It was one big party, which I thought was great! It was during this time that I first did cocaine. It was my usual pattern — I didn't feel high at first, but I imitated what everyone else did who was using, pretending to be high.

I returned to school only long enough to save money, drop out, and move West. As a part of the move, a friend and I decided to write a book of our adventure entitled, *America by Cars & Bars*. We planned to describe the countryside with special emphasis on the best bars along the way. We did a lot of research! Our route was planned around distilleries and breweries. About halfway across the country, we were drinking so much we were unable to remember enough of the bars to write about them. After visiting a particularly large distillery, we had to abandon the project entirely.

We looked up a friend of mine from my summer hotel job. This man was much older than we were, very alcoholic, and in and out of jail a lot. He let us stay with him, which was okay at first, but before long, he started using heroin and drinking heavily. Time after time, I bailed him out, took him to detox, and covered the bounced checks he wrote. This went on for two years. Finally, a nurse in a detox told me to "let go and let God," to "detach with love," and to take care of myself for once. I was 19 years old, but felt 119 years old.

I took her advice and moved 500 miles away. I believed the move would change everything. I thought I could be different. Soon my loneliness led me to a group of familiar-acting people. After a few beers we were the best of friends. I fell in love with a man who used a variety of drugs, especially cocaine. I was so happy, I asked him to marry me the night we met. As we went through my savings, I experienced blackouts. It never occurred to me that maybe I had met a clone of the guy I'd just left.

When another guy I knew wanted to borrow my car and found out he couldn't, he attacked us with a baseball bat. Some people might have called the police, but our choice was to buy a rifle. We drove to his house and started shooting at him and everyone in it. I know today that it was God's work that no one got hit by the bullets.

I freaked out in jail, after learning there was no bail set and my charge was attempted murder. I called my brother, who, against my wishes, informed my mother of my predicament. Four days later, all charges were dropped and I was released. Later, when I came into C.A. and heard people talking about a Higher Power, then heard the *Footprints* poem, I remembered this situation and the miraculous dropping of all charges. I knew then that God had been with me the whole time, that He carried me through those times I felt so alone and so scared, and that it was God who protected those people from getting hit by the bullets.

When I got out of jail, instead of leaving that crazy life, I continued my insane way of living. I was on the run for the next three years. We did geographic moves from coast-to-coast, escaping warrants and usually staying one step ahead of the law. Sometimes, however, we didn't manage to stay one step ahead and would do jail time for some burglary or other sloppy crime. The bars I had started to write about before, turned out to be prison bars. I was left alone a lot and felt abandoned. I didn't know my boyfriend had the disease of addiction and that the disease was what made him do the things he did to get high. I only knew that I didn't come first and felt that he didn't love me. But I believed that if I were good, he would stay with me.

My family had no idea where I was during these years. I would occasionally call collect and say everything was great. Deep down inside, however, I was a scared little girl who was afraid to come home for fear of being considered a failure.

We held up stores, ripped off hitchhikers, slept in cars and shelters, stole from churches, and sold our blood. We did all this to get money for drugs and alcohol. I felt my needs were not important. I went without food so my boyfriend could get high. I cried a lot, always wanting to die. I knew no way out of this insanity. I didn't reach out for help.

At one point, an old friend rescued and nursed me back to semi-health. She sent me back to my mom's house and to this day, I don't recall how I got there.

I was devastated living without my boyfriend. I ached to return to him and that lifestyle. After six months, he came to me and we tried to make it work again. History repeated itself. We led a normal life for a few months, until we met up with a cocaine dealer. That was the beginning of the end. I resumed the enabler role, covering the bad checks, the stolen credit cards, and the people he'd ripped off. After living this way for many years, I had no self-esteem and no self-worth. The desire to stop living got stronger.

The turning point came when he committed a large burglary, then brought the stolen items and a stolen car across state lines. I was subpoenaed to testify against him in the case, and faced my own jail time if I didn't show up in court. I was afraid of facing my boyfriend in court and testifying against him. I now believe God did for me what I could not do for myself. My boyfriend jumped bail, so no court appearance was ever required of me. Since that time, I've seen him only once, when I visited him where he was hiding out. I wanted to die like I never had before. I drank and did as much cocaine as I could for the next two years. Sometimes my old boyfriend would call; I would tell him what I was doing, hoping he'd say he'd come back, but he never did.

I wanted to stop using cocaine, but every day I had to get high. I started my day with it; I couldn't breathe without it. Everything and everybody in my life involved cocaine. I lived the life of a vampire, going out only after dark, and crawling into my bed when the sun rose. I didn't do anything anymore except get high (or low, as I refer to it today).

One night I went to bed crying that I wanted to stop using cocaine. The dealer was in my room. He told me that I should really get help if I wanted to stop that badly.

That night I prayed out loud to God for help. I was depressed. I believed that I didn't have long to go before my heart gave out or my brain exploded.

The very next day at work, a coworker came in like he always did. However, this particular day, he seemed to be glowing as he crossed the room. Suddenly, I remembered he'd been court-ordered to attend Cocaine Anonymous meetings. I thought he might have information that would help me. Today I believe that he was a direct answer to my prayers of the night before. Because I always made it to work, no one else there knew I was in trouble. But this guy had noticed the bags under my eyes, and that I didn't bathe regularly or do laundry, though he never said anything about my deteriorating condition. This particular day we talked; he told me about a C.A. meeting that coming Friday night and offered to take me. Each day I asked him if he would still take me, and he said that he would. When Friday came, he told me he couldn't take me after all, but by then, I had some belief that I would get help at this meeting.

I gathered all the courage I had inside and went to the meeting alone. I remember that my legs felt as if they weighed 500 pounds apiece as I walked towards the meeting room. There seemed to be 100 people there. They were all laughing and smiling. I sure wasn't laughing or smiling, and hadn't for some time. The chairperson read the Preamble and asked if there were any newcomers. Somehow, I raised my hand. I rambled on about my situation and that I wanted to stop using cocaine but couldn't. A bunch of people told me to "keep coming back" and gave me their phone numbers after the meeting.

I haven't used cocaine since that meeting. I wore C.A. like a shield when people from my old life came around. I lived in the same house for my first six months of recovery, despite people using cocaine around me. I clung to the Program with all my might. I came home from meetings and wrote about the topic or the speaker. I read the Twelve and Twelve. I asked God for help with the cravings and dreams that came along after stopping.

I continued to drink for another five to six months and stayed connected to my old life. I was half-stepping in and out of the C.A. Fellowship. I couldn't understand why my life didn't get any better! Each time I drank, I felt worse.

Eventually, I made a commitment to myself to live a sober life, one day at a time. I started attending Step study meetings, got a sponsor and began to get honest with myself. I had told everyone that I had been sober from the time I stopped using cocaine, but that wasn't true. I had to humble myself and tell my newfound friends that I'd been drinking the whole time. I had to tell them that my real sobriety date was six months later than they thought.

I began to see what situations triggered the urge to get high and drink. I learned about myself, what makes me happy and unhappy. When I began listening to others' stories and identifying with their feelings, I could see that yes, I was also an alcoholic.

Once, in a meeting, the word "insanity" came up. My whole life began to make sense. I'd always tried to make sense out of an insane situation! I began to learn about this disease that I have. It is a progressive disease and it will never go away. I heard once in a meeting that while we're in a meeting getting better, the disease is out in the parking lot doing push-ups and wind sprints, getting stronger! It is patient and cunning. I know today that its sole purpose is to kill me, whether instantly or by slow death.

People understand and love me in the rooms of C.A. I don't need to explain myself or justify my actions. They loved me when I could not love myself. All I had to do was show up. They told me it was okay to screw up, that this was a program of "progress, not perfection." The words to "How It Works" suddenly made sense to me. I have learned, though slowly, to ask for help when I need it. Those feelings of hopelessness and loneliness have gone away. It didn't happen overnight; but then, I didn't get to the state I was in overnight, either.

So, while I didn't dream of becoming a drug addict when I was that little girl, becoming an addict led me to Cocaine Anonymous. C.A. is the only thing that is helping me to grow up and become the person I was meant to be. For that, I am grateful.

4

THE GREAT PRETENDER

This addict spent so much time trying to fool others, that it took recovery to make him realize the only person he was fooling was himself.

*T*LEARNED EARLY in life to pretend I was something, somewhere, or someone that I wasn't. As I think about it, that old fifties R & B tune *The Great Pretender* comes to mind.

In the back of a limousine at the cemetery on the day of my mother's funeral and interment, my older brother shook me hard to wake me, though I wasn't asleep. I was pretending because I didn't want to be my father's crutch as he staggered to the grave. Ol' Dad wasn't pretending; he was dead drunk.

Why did Dad prefer the bottle to his family? Before my mother's death, he was always drunk, but without an excuse. After she died, my father's best friend and constant companion wasn't a person, it was a bottle.

A few months after my mother's death, he was handed another reason to drink when my brothers and I were shipped off to live with relatives. So what was it that my father liked so much about being drunk? I just had to find out.

I remember very little about the first drink because it led to a second and a third. Before my friends and I had finished, we had drunk a quart of vodka and a couple of bottles of cheap wine. Somehow, we found ourselves at the entrance of a hospital, because two of us had decided we were insane and needed help. We were met by a guard who took us to a small room to process us for admission, or so I thought. Actually, he had called the police. While we were waiting, I got impatient and told the guard that if he didn't get us some help, my friend might just pull a gun and shoot him.

Evidently, the man must have taken me seriously, even though I was pretending, because he had my friend stand up. As the guard began his search, my friend pulled a small-caliber pistol from his coat pocket. As he tried to hand the weapon to the startled guard, a skirmish took place and the guard ended up beneath him. It wasn't what my friend had intended. He was only pretending; the gun wasn't even loaded.

The judge gave me a choice: suspended jail sentence and probation or move and live with my brother. It wasn't much of a choice to me, but I relocated. I hoped a fresh start and new friends were all I needed to become a law-abiding citizen.

I consumed large quantities of cocaine in my new location. The drug was first given to me by a well-meaning, but misguided friend. He also happened to be a pharmacist in possession of several bottles of the real stuff. Back in those days, 1970 give or take a year, I had to beg people to get high with me. It may have been the geographic location or the quality of the powder, but every time I snorted the stuff, I always ended up barricading myself and whoever was there with me until what we had was snorted or flushed.

Things didn't get much better. One day, I had an unexpected visit from a U.S. marshal. He had a five-count indictment in his possession with my name on it. While I was pretending to be cool, the charges ranging from sales to conspiracy to distribute cocaine, were read. All I could say to myself was, "Are we having fun yet?" I had visualized this moment, when the law would finally catch up with me, for years. I had thought it would be a little more exciting, full of gunplay and blood and guts. That was nothing like what really happened. I signed on the dotted line, where it indicated that I understood the charges against me and told me when to appear for arraignment. Before I even had a chance to change my mind or fabricate another story, the marshal was finished.

I hit my knees and for the first time I asked God (if there was one) to HELP ME! Within twenty-four hours I was a patient in a hospital that had a whole floor full of crazies just like me. I was taken there by a friend, in fact, the guy who gave me my first shot of coke. He assured me that this was a place where I could rest. I needed a lot of rest because I was delusional. (My plans were to head south into Mexico or Latin America. There I would find the cave where all the lost souls were being held captive and couldn't become human again until I fought and killed their captor.)

Needless to say my friend lied to me. I got no rest. But I did acquire a few tools I thought would help me later on. All this rhetoric about having to stop using drugs, especially cocaine, made me really skeptical. I hadn't come to this place to get straight. I'd come here for rest and to escape the pressure state and federal agents were putting on me to cooperate. During our only meeting, these fellas offered me this terrific deal — cooperate or go to prison. I needed a place where I could sort all of this out without distraction and without a warrant. I was told that the law couldn't touch me...until I was discharged.

All this time, the folks at the hospital were trying to get it through my thick skull that I had to accept responsibility for my own actions. Hey, I had a list a mile long of people I blamed. It began with my mother, who died on me when I was too young, a father who loved booze more than he loved me, and a pharmacist who wanted help doing his drug of choice. It included all the folks who came to love the "White Lady" so much that they gave me vast sums of money (and I.O.U.s) to go back and get more of her from a connection who was only too glad to sell part of her for cash and the rest on account. Sure, it was all my fault. While we are checking this list of people who were responsible for the sad state of my life, let's not forget my wife. She was utterly shocked to find out from my counselor that I was a cocaine addict. She thought that during all those years of active using I'd had a bad cold. About the only thing that was cold in our marriage was my side of the bed.

During my days of rage, I was in love with many women. However, being insane, the affairs were somewhat predictable and would go something like this: I would meet a woman. That very night I would discover she was the One I'd been looking for all of my life. Both of us were loving people: she loved my cocaine, and I loved her body. When I ran out of cocaine, she would run out on me. I'd be depressed for a couple of days. Eventually, I'd wipe my eyes sufficiently to hide any trace of a broken heart, pick myself up, and go home to my wife.

Being the Great Pretender, I thought I had everyone fooled into thinking that I had fully accepted this recovery stuff, everyone except the drunk who facilitated my First Step. He waited patiently while I told my small group the gory details of a promising life gone bad. When I had finished, I thought the old fart would give me a hug and advise me to write a book. Instead, he got real irritated and said he was pissed off because I had wasted his time. He said that anyone who had a best friend die in his arms while on guard duty in Vietnam without showing any feeling about it would use again and probably die of an overdose. His comments really angered me. Oh, sure, I would probably use again, and maybe even die. But what really hacked me off was his insight. He saw through my act; the Great Pretender didn't fool him one bit.

I eventually got over my anger. I reasoned with myself that it was silly to get worked-up over something that never even happened. I mean, the closest I ever got to guard duty in 'Nam was using the typewriter to make up the roster of those guys who would risk their lives to protect me and my real best friend, who wasn't even a person. It was a plant! It was a bag of opium-laced marijuana. Until I met a new Lady a few years later, Mary Jane and I were the very best of friends.

After my release from the treatment center, it took me a while to find the right meeting to attend. At one meeting I was told that the function of the group was to help alcoholics, that it neither wanted to know nor hear about any drug problems. I knew this was home sweet home. I figured that as long as I didn't use alcohol, I could smoke all the pot and shoot all the coke I wanted yet still be a member in good standing with the group.

By the time I celebrated my first year of "sobriety," I had made all my court appearances, pled guilty to one of the charges, and been sentenced to a four-year term in a federal correctional institution. My "first" birthday was a real tearjerker. Being the Great Pretender, I told the group that I was crying because I had never been accepted by so many for just being myself. But I was really crying because I had to go to prison while they got to stay home and talk about their alcoholic lives. Even the joint I smoked on the way home after the meeting did little to improve my mood.

I will always remember the day my brother took me to prison. I was cool on the plane ride, in the rented car, during the walk to the entrance, even after the farewell hug. I didn't lose it until I went through the big metal door. At the last minute, I remember my brother telling me that he would give me a couple of dollars until my funds were posted. I grabbed the door and attempted to turn the handle. I then discovered that while it was relatively easy to get into this place, it was going to be another, altogether different matter, to get out again. This was also a very special day for another reason — it was the last day I ever used any mind-bending drugs.

Recovery meetings were available, and I tried a few of them. But, with a guard present at all of the get-togethers "for our protection," I was afraid to reveal anything about myself. So, I took advantage of the other rehabilitation programs.

I started running around the track, up to six miles a day. The track was one place where I could be alone to collect my thoughts, process my beliefs, and experience some constructive self-dialogue. As my body and mind responded to the new habit of long-distance running, I became more positive and assertive.

It has been said that in every experience is a lesson. During my incarceration I learned many. Certainly the one I still carry with me today is the discovery that there really is one Presence and one Power — That which I choose to call God. By relaxing and becoming still in mind and body, I was eventually able to make my own conscious connection with this Presence and Power. As soon as I had become somewhat consistent in this practice, I shared my insight with anyone who would listen. Sometime later, I would learn that these were Steps Eleven and Twelve in the recovery program, and that they were at the end, not at the beginning of the process.

By the time I was paroled, the seeds of a spiritually centered life had been planted and nurtured. I was being led in thought, as well as action, to the irresistible conclusion of what was, in truth, my birthright: a good life filled with positive relationships, exceptional health, and rewarding prosperity.

Outside the gate, I stumbled and nearly fell, but through the grace of God, I was able to catch myself. At this most vulnerable time, I was directed by angels, who appeared as mere mortals, to the Fellowship of Cocaine Anonymous. Attending meetings has become an integral part of my life, as important to my well-being as breathing. In my personal program of recovery, I am developing an intuitive ability to see past the appearance of others and into their hearts. It is there that I find what I have discovered in myself — the Presence and Power that guides us to our greatest good, to be one in all and to know all is One.

The last time I consciously pretended to be someone I was not was in prison. The place was filled with Great Pretenders. I was shocked to discover that of all the criminals doing time, I was one of the very few who admitted his guilt. Almost everyone else there faithfully defended his innocence. Talk about pretending! Right then and there I hung up the masks.

Not until a few months ago did it occur to me that I could be a pretender again. In a few weeks I will be a member of a summer stock theater group at a local university. I was really excited when I read the script of one play and found the perfect part: a practicing alcoholic, chain-smoker, who throws matches out of windows and commands trees to die. No such luck. The director gave me the part of a stuffy, narrow-minded businessman, the type who makes all the right moves. That's going to be a real challenge.

What excites me about all of this is my new insight. Before, I was a Great Pretender to protect myself so others wouldn't see the real me. Now I am the real me who can slip into a character, get on stage, and have a wonderful time, giving a delightful gift that before had been abused — the Great Pretender.

Last year I was married for the second time. My wife, being a kindergarten teacher, knows well how to treat children my age. The best part of our relationship is that we share common interests and have a mutual respect for life.

My prayer for everyone is visual. I see all around me the peace of mind and serenity of heart that surpasses all understanding. Accepting it makes it so.

5

THE LAWYER'S PLEA

This lawyer's prayer to a Higher Power she didn't even believe in brought her a reprieve from a life sentence of addiction, and gave her a new outlook on life.

I AM A woman, a lawyer in my early forties living in a suburb of a major city, where my cat and I share a condo. I am presently more than five years sober. I am happy with myself and my life almost all of the time now.

When I came to the program of Cocaine Anonymous, I was not very happy with myself or my life. I had not been for as long as I could remember. I was virtually a failed suicide. I was driven to the Program when I discovered that I could not use enough cocaine to die.

Things started out differently for me as a child. I was bright and full of promise; a sunny, yellow-haired little girl who was liked by teachers and labelled precocious. In retrospect, though, it seems that this thing I now call "the disease" was always with me.

Among my classmates and friends, I always felt somehow defective or flawed. Though I looked okay on the outside, I felt worthless, inept, and bad. I stayed away from others so they wouldn't find out who I really was inside. I did well in classes and always tried to dress exactly right, in hopes of feeling better inside by looking better outside. This never worked for long.

I went to college at the end of the drug-saturated sixties. I smoked as much pot, drank as much beer, and ate as much acid as I could get my hands on. The first clue I should have noticed relating to the nature of my disease occurred at the end of my first year in college. I went to the house of a pot dealer in the next town and found a group around the kitchen table. I asked what they were doing. They said, "Heroin," to which I replied without hesitation, "Gimme some!"

Although I knew that heroin was an addictive drug and that people died from it regularly, this knowledge had no impact on me. With the first opportunity, my disease took control. I would go to any length to alter my consciousness, get away from the noise in my head, be anywhere but inside my skin, or be anyone but myself.

My love affair with heroin lasted five years. It took me through forty-odd states, a couple of minor arrests, a marriage, and a divorce. I also had a child, a little girl, who was unwittingly carried along on this odyssey; a miniature hostage of my addiction.

I worked as a journalist, a stripper, a barmaid, and a prostitute. Prostitution paid the best, so I stuck with it — quite a position for a middle-class girl from the suburbs! None of it was too high a price to pay. If I had been able to seriously look at my life, I might have concluded that staying anesthetized wasn't worth the pain it was causing. This was a dilemma I resolved by staying loaded; therefore never being able to take a look at it.

After about five years, the "heroin period" abruptly came to a halt. I overdosed for about the hundredth time. This time my friends couldn't bring me around. The paramedics took me to a hospital, where the emergency room doctors revived me and released me; they didn't have much drug treatment in hospitals at that time.

I realized that heroin didn't work for me anymore. I had discovered the phenomenon of tolerance; the amount required now to get me high was more than the amount that would kill me.

So I went dry. I went into therapy. I went back to college. In a compulsive fashion, I worked my outcall business, raised a child, made honors, and graduated college in three years. I thought that achievement and material success would bring me happiness, self-esteem, and contentment.

After college I married well. We had money, cars, a condo, and charge accounts. I got a good and challenging job. My daughter was well-settled. I was not using. I was miserable and didn't know why. I had everything that was supposed to work, but I was still quietly dying inside and filled with self-loathing. I didn't know then that I was still suffering from untreated drug addiction, even when I was dry.

I met Sister Cocaine a couple of years later. My best thinking told me that this would be different and, for a while, it was. My husband and I snorted socially on weekends. After a few months, I noticed that he and I were different. He could go to bed with most of the bag still there! He could save some of the stuff for another day or even another week! I used as much as I could get my hands on, whenever I could get it.

I went to law school then, and stayed virtually dry for three years while I immersed myself in classes, then the Bar exam. I thought I didn't really have a problem, despite my old experience with heroin, because I could always put it down when something important enough came up.

After the Bar exam, my cocaine use resumed and increased dramatically. An occasional indulgence quickly became a nightly ritual. I was locked in the bedroom in a drug-induced paranoid state every night by 7 P.M. or 8 P.M. I tried to limit the amount I used per day and to take days off from using, but the amounts and frequency increased, and the unmanageability of my behavior increased as well.

I was able to obtain a job as a lawyer, but the marriage was over. My by-then-teenaged daughter finally left my home in disgust. I was soon fired from the lawyer job, which I could no longer handle. I got a less-demanding job with flexible hours, so I could work around my drug use.

I soon found myself with two roommates sharing a cheap, one-bedroom apartment. We were all working and also dealing, but we still had trouble paying the rent. Every night, I came home and got so loaded by 7 P.M. that I was hearing voices outside coming to get me. My nights were filled with sweating terror, crawling on the floor of the dark apartment so "they" wouldn't see me. Every morning I swore not to do that much again, but the next night was always the same.

Ultimately, in despair, I called the Cocaine Anonymous hotline. I was sure it wouldn't work for me, but I had no one else to call. I tried a few meetings, but came home and got high afterwards. I didn't pay any attention to suggestions of "90 meetings in 90 days." The suggestion of prayer was inconceivable to me. I didn't think I believed in God, and I was sure God didn't believe in me.

I went on this way, getting loaded and attending meetings intermittently, for about six months. No one, least of all me, thought I could actually get sober. One night, near dawn, after hours of abject and pitiful terror, and crawling on the floor, I got desperate enough to try anything. I invented a simplistic form of the Third Step prayer. I knelt on the floor, folded my hands, and said: "God, if You are up there — and I don't think You are — if You give a damn about me — and I don't think You do — please take this thing from me and I will do anything You want for the rest of my life." With that, a feeling of warmth and peace came over me, and I lay down and serenely went to sleep.

It has been several years since that day. The obsession to use has never returned. I pray every day and every night, on my knees, thanking God for another day, and asking for guidance and strength.

After I was "struck sober," I was still insane; I had been before I ever used. I got a sponsor and worked Steps Four and Five in the first few months, with some improvement, but my self-loathing persisted. The committee in my head criticized my every move and called me names from morning to night.

My first sponsor moved. A second one was put in front of me after I prayed for one. I worked through the Steps with this second sponsor, and again with the next. With each successive trip through the Steps, more has been revealed. My life has steadily become more serene and peaceful.

I have been entrusted with various commitments; from coffee person, to meeting secretary, to answering the hotline. Each of these commitments has contributed to my growth in sobriety. The experience of sponsorship has been the most rewarding, as I get to share in the miracle of recovery and growth with the women who have been placed in my life.

Today I like myself, deeply, from the inside out. My fear of people has been greatly reduced and continues to shrink. The areas of personal relations, daily life, and work are calm and pleasant; no longer chaotic. I enjoy the friendship of my now adult daughter and my parents.

It has taken several years of work, patience, hope, love, inventories, tears, and honest sharing of feelings to get to this point. It would never have happened without the courage and faith I learned in the program of Cocaine Anonymous, and the Steps to guide me in cleaning up the wreckage of my past and re-establishing relations.

Today, in my life, there is a feeling of peace and security such as I have never known. Life seems good to me today. I haven't felt the self-loathing or the screaming, ragged pain in my guts at all for a couple of years now, thanks to the Steps and the healing brought about by working them.

I know that I am a different, much better person now than I ever was, even before I used. All of the Promises have come true in my life. Each day sober is better than the one before, in a lot of ways.

Today I know that I am powerless over the outcome of everything and that my life is still unmanageable by me. Today I believe that a Power greater than myself can, and is, restoring me to sanity in every area of my life. I have faith that this miracle will continue, as long as I keep doing the footwork.

I wish that everyone could find what has been given to me. But I know that only a few will be willing enough to take this path. I hope and pray that you, my reader, will be one of those. I lost nothing but my misery.

6

HE THOUGHT HE HAD CONTROL

It only took one person carrying the message at the right time to give him the hope, strength, and courage to go on.

*M*Y LIFE GOT to be about as unmanageable as possible, before I took some action to get help from someone for my addiction. Let me give you a little history of my mind-altering substances use, and how I got to where I am today.

When I was about twelve years old, I started drinking. I didn't start drinking because I really liked to. I did it to be like everyone else, "a part of." It was also a way to feel more grown up, the same reason that I started smoking cigarettes. I've never been able to drink very much without getting sick, but that never stopped me from drinking. I just learned to accept the fact that if I was going to get blitzed, I was going to get sick, too.

When I was thirteen, I hung around some guys who were sniffing glue. Not wanting to be different, when they offered me some, I accepted. That was my first drug abuse. I probably only did glue for about a month or two, but I did it on a pretty regular basis. I used to have blackouts and come out of them in the strangest places. It used to scare me. I quit that drug when my mom moved to the other side of the state. It was a real small midwestern country town, so I pretty much did what was the norm: I drank.

Once I turned eighteen, I moved in with my uncle for the first few months or so, then got an apartment with my cousin. I went out with a girl one night, and she broke out a little baggie full of pot. I had never seen that stuff; I had only heard of it from people who didn't have a clue. When the joint passed my way, there was no way I was going to look like a fool and say no.

Nope, I spent the night with her laughing and having a great time. I laughed at just about anything that was said, even when nothing was said at all. You know what? I never got sick either! Yes, marijuana was to become my drug of choice.

For the next seventeen years, I used marijuana on a daily basis. I hung around with the drug crowd because they liked me for what I was: a drug user. I also loved the way drugs made me feel. It was as if I could face anything that came my way, as long as I had my drugs. I got married at 21 and had two children by the time I was 23. I got up each day and went to work to support my family. But when it was time to relax, it was time for a bud — and I don't mean a beer.

About the time I was 26, I met some new friends through a job change who took me away from the friends I used to associate with. These new friends liked to do cocaine. When it was offered to me, of course I wanted to check it out. I had already been arrested once before for possession of marijuana with the intent to sell. I could never afford to buy drugs in the amount that I liked to use them. I learned right off that if I sold enough, I could get mine free. All my friends used drugs, so it only made sense that if they were going to buy drugs from someone they might as well buy them from me.

About six months into my cocaine abuse, I got laid off. My wife was beginning to scare me with her abuse of cocaine, yet I couldn't see how my own abuse was affecting me. We made a series of geographics to escape the cocaine. I had never done a drug that took control of me so quickly. My marriage continued to decline, although I didn't really notice it. I still continued to smoke my pot and was unaware of what was happening around me.

One day my wife woke up and said that she couldn't take it anymore: she was leaving me. For the next year, I was pretty much alone. I started to get out and date after a year. That's when my drug use started to increase again. I was back in circulation.

A friend of mine started to sell cocaine and was making big money. I was envious, but hesitant to start selling again for fear of another arrest. I figured, though, that if I only sold to my closest friends, I wouldn't get busted.

It didn't take but about a week or two before I started snorting coke in small amounts, telling myself that I could do this as long as I didn't do very much. Yeah, right! That didn't last long either. I did so much that my face would hurt. I tried to pretend that I had a cold; that this was the reason I was always sniffling.

I was soon introduced to freebasing. At first it was something new, and I had fun with it. But very soon afterwards, I realized that this was one drug I was going to have a lot of problems with. The very first time I tried freebasing, I couldn't bring myself to leave the house where the rock was. The whole night I kept saying that I had to go, but it was like I was in a trance. I just couldn't leave as long as there was some left. After that, I tried to stay away from my friend's house. I was really afraid of that drug and its controlling effect on me.

It wasn't long before I was making freebase at my house, thinking I could control the amount I used if only I could control the amount I cooked up. I made it in colors: red, blue, and green. That way I wouldn't mistake ceiling for fallen pieces of rock cocaine. This worked for awhile, but then everything on the floor appeared to be red, blue, and green.

My bottom was getting closer every day. I spent all of my time in my bedroom, because that's where I made and sold my drugs. I smoked it there with a few friends, because I had kids at home and didn't want them to know I was freebasing cocaine. I was becoming aware that I was not only ruining my life, but was also starting to bring a lot of other people down with me.

One day I called the owner of the company I was working

41

for at that time. I told him that I was having a problem with cocaine; that I needed some time off to go into a hospital or get some help with my problem. He told me that he was glad that I talked with him and that he understood. He also told me to take all the time I needed to take care of my problem; that my job would be waiting for me when I came back.

To the addict that I was, this was like a free pass to do all the partying I wanted. Now I didn't have to worry about losing my job, because my boss said to take all the time that I needed.

By this time, I did not leave my house at all. For dinner, I would either send my kids out, or have someone else bring it in. It was easy to get someone to do anything for me as long as they thought they were going to get some rock out of it. I was basing every waking hour by then. The time between my waking and sleeping was getting longer and longer. I lived like that for about two months. I had developed all the symptoms of paranoia. You know, like when you are sure there are people outside in the bushes watching you (the "bush people"). I had also started to believe that everyone was using me to get my drugs. It got to the point I couldn't even understand my own thinking. I felt like I was totally out of control, and I was right.

During the last two months of my using, my ex-wife admitted herself into a chemical dependency unit and stayed for a three-day detox. She was only out of there three days when she readmitted herself for a thirty-day program.

My ex-wife called me once while she was in the hospital and asked me if I was going to get help. I weighed close to 140 pounds and looked terrible; my normal weight is 180 pounds. I told her that I would get help when she got out of the hospital, but that for now I had no one to take care of the kids.

When my ex-wife had been out of the hospital for about a week, she told me that I could now go into the hospital, as she would take care of the kids. I told her, "Yeah, this weekend I will," though I knew in my mind I probably wouldn't. That Friday you might say that an intervention was done on me. Actually, it was more like an interception. I was busted by the police. They broke down my door, held me at gunpoint, handcuffed me, and proceeded to tear apart my house. I'm glad my kids were in school at the time. They were saved from witnessing my humiliation. That night, with the help of my ex-wife, I bailed myself out of jail.

My "sort-of girlfriend" at the time came over. She was going to stay with me for moral support, I guess. Remember though, that I had been in jail for about seven hours, and by then I was jonesing. I called one of my connections and told him to bring over what he owed me. My girlfriend told me that if I smoked that stuff after what I had just gone through, she was leaving me. You probably know what I said to her: "Goodbye!"

My friend brought the coke over. I couldn't talk him into staying and smoking it with me. He was too busy, or maybe just paranoid. At any rate, I was all alone. I did an amount in fifteen minutes that used to last me all night. I was at my bottom; I couldn't get a hit big enough. I was feeling worse than I had ever felt in my life. I didn't care if I lived or died. I didn't know what to do.

I got on the phone and asked my ex-wife if she would take me to the treatment center. She told me that she would take me there in the morning because they couldn't admit me until then.

I was admitted into the hospital on a Saturday morning. They weren't sure if my insurance would cover me for the thirty-day program or just the three-day detox. They said they would let me know on Monday, after my insurance office opened.

I spent Saturday and Sunday in kind of a daze, detoxing. I don't really recall what went on, except that I ate a lot of food and felt safe from using.

When Monday came, I got the news that I could only stay for the three days of detox, and I would be released the next morning. The counselor there could see that I was starting to panic. He had me sit in on a couple of group sessions with the other patients. That night I couldn't sleep. I was so afraid that when I got out of the hospital I would start using again. I was positive that I had no self-control, and I remembered that my ex-wife had come into this same place for three days and was out using within a week. I felt doomed.

As I sat on my bed, about one o'clock in the morning, the nurse on the graveyard shift came in to see what my problem was. With tears in my eyes, I proceeded to tell her how I felt. I didn't know it then, but she was my light at the end of the tunnel, where only a few minutes before there had been total darkness. She shared with me that she was a recovering addict. She told me that not everyone needed to enter a chemical dependency unit for 30 days or, for that matter, any days to stay sober. She told me to go to a meeting when I got out the next morning, and to just not use for that day.

The next morning, when I was being released, the counselor told me that he would like me to come to aftercare on Wednesday night. I told him that I would be there, and was off to my first meeting right then.

Going to my first Twelve Step meeting was a scary thing for me to do. The place was an old building, and the people didn't look like anyone I wanted to be friends with. But I was there on a mission. The mission was to stop using drugs so I could get on with my life.

I stood up and said that I was an addict and an alcoholic. I didn't think I was an alcoholic, but I thought that if I didn't admit to it, they wouldn't let me stay. I started going to work, coming home, eating dinner, and rushing off to a meeting every day. I didn't know what I was doing, but the people kept saying things like: "Keep coming back" and "Sit down, shut up, and listen." So I did. I found Cocaine Anonymous after about a week of sobriety. Right away I knew that this was where I belonged. The people there did drugs the way I did, and I could relate to that. I wasn't sober long enough to relate to sobriety; it was the drug-a-logues that kept me interested.

Slowly but surely, I started hearing other messages like: "Get a sponsor and work the Steps or you're probably going to go back out and use again." I had a hard time choosing a sponsor. Nobody seemed right for me. I thought I was so different from everyone else. Boy, was I wrong.

I was in a meeting one night, feeling that everyone there knew I didn't have a sponsor yet and wasn't working a program the way they say you're supposed to. You know — that feeling of not being a part of the Program. Well, it was making my life really uncomfortable. I decided that I was choosing a sponsor at this meeting no matter what. You see, in the short time I had been in the Program, I had learned that my best thinking wasn't the best thing that had ever happened to me. As the meeting was ending and everyone was getting up to leave, I closed my eyes, turned around, and asked the first male in front of me to be my sponsor. I know now that he was more unsure of being my sponsor than I was of picking him.

What I've learned is to take a little direction and not be so much of a know-it-all. I've worked the Steps with my sponsor to the best of my ability. He has taught me not to worry about getting a grade on them. If I don't like the way I did them, I can always do them again, and I have.

I've been of service ever since I got a sponsor, because that's what he told me would keep me sober. He also gave me his coffee commitment. I've been a literature person, secretary, and hotline phone person. I have my own panel at a hospital, and I'm chairperson at another facility. I continue to be of service for the Program, because I know that I can only get out of it what I put into it. It has always been there for me.

I did some time in jail after being eleven months sober, as a result of the charges brought against me when I was arrested, but you know what? It was okay. God let me have a little time under my belt before he let me go into jail. By then I was well into the recovery part of this Program and wouldn't have had it any other way. I was of service to the Program in jail, too. They have panels come in to share their experience, strength, and hope. Thank God for that because it helped keep me focused on where I was trying to take my life.

I met my present wife in the Program. Today I'm a happily married man. We go to a lot of C.A. functions. We learned to do things in sobriety that we never did before. I've learned to roller-skate, water-ski, snow-ski, and just recently, how to dance with my wife. Some people may already know how to do these things, but I was always too cool to make a fool of myself trying to learn them. Today I've learned that I can face my fears and walk through them. I'm really proud of having the courage to go out on the dance floor and fast-dance. My wife loves to dance. I always felt bad when she would ask me to dance, and I would say no because I couldn't overcome my fear of getting out there. When things like this happen to me, I know I'm growing because I'm doing something about it.

I don't want you to think that everything is perfect in my life today; it's not, but it's a lot better than it was when I used drugs. Today I have real friends that don't want something from me for their friendship. Today I'm not the same way I used to be. I'm still the same person, but now I'm someone who enjoys life and tries to put something into it instead of seeing what I can get out of it. That's a whole different life for me.

This Program is not for people who need it; rather, it's for people who want it. Believe me — I want it!

To anyone who reads this, and can relate to my story and the feelings being shared, I can honestly say: no matter how bad things look at times during sobriety, they get better. And no matter how good things are, they can get worse. That's called life, and living it on life's terms is what the Program is about. As long as I accept life as being exactly the way it's supposed to be, I'm pretty comfortable with myself. When it's not going my way and I'm not accepting the way things are, I'm usually miserable. I have a choice today: to accept and be happy, or to not accept and be miserable. Most of all, I can choose to do the footwork to change my life; because no one is able to do it for me.

Cocaine Anonymous gave me back my life. As far as I'm concerned, the only gram in town for me is the Program.

7

"NICE" GIRLS GET ADDICTED, TOO

*She never thought it could happen to her, but she discovered the hard way
that crack cocaine doesn't care who you are.*

*U*NLIKE MANY OF the stories I've heard from
other addicts, my family life and growing-up years
were nothing short of wonderful. My loving parents did their best to provide a healthy, comfortable environment for us three kids. I was the middle child, with an older
sister and a younger brother. My mom was a superb full-time
homemaker who excelled at all domestic tasks, from baking to
needlework. My dad supported us, working at the same
company from before my birth until he retired. He *never* took
a day off work unless it was a scheduled vacation or he was too
sick to get out of bed, which was very, very rare.

As far as drugs or alcohol went, we always had liquor in the
house, but it was only served when company came to visit
around the holidays, or on special occasions. Illegal drugs
were never even close to being an issue. I think the strongest
thing we ever had in the house was cough syrup with codeine.
Although my mother only rarely sipped a glass of wine or a
weak highball, my father enjoyed himself during the periodic
instances when it became permissible to drink. Generally
speaking, he got drunk. Much later in life, with the help of the
Program, I am now able to recognize his alcoholic behavior
patterns. But back then, all I could see was that when he drank,
he got happy and funny, and he made me laugh a lot.

Since I have come into recovery and have learned about my
disease, I strongly believe that I was born with a predisposi-
tion toward addiction and began exhibiting addictive behavior long before I ever started doing drugs. I learned to lie at

the same time I learned to talk. I always felt the need to twist the truth about things I did or what happened in my life, usually for no other reason than to make myself look better. Petty thievery was also one of my regular habits, including, but not limited to taking cash from my parents, minor shoplifting, and pretty much anything else I thought I could get away with.

In spite of these character defects, my childhood was relatively sane and normal. I spent eight years in the Girl Scouts, made friends easily, and did well in school. I relate this only to show that you don't have to come from an unhappy or dysfunctional home to wind up an addict. Our disease is non-discriminatory, and it can happen to anyone.

I was not introduced to drugs until my senior year in high school. Marijuana, being the first, triggered an instantaneous love affair. No matter what activity I was involved with, pot made me feel like it was more fun. I distinctly remember thinking that I could enjoy doing anything if I were stoned. Soon other kinds of drugs such as THC, mescaline, and reds began to surface in my circle of friends. I experimented with all of them; uppers or downers, it made no difference, as long as I "copped a buzz."

For the most part, during my using career, I was capable of functioning in a fairly normal fashion. The secretarial skills I acquired in high school earned me a government job that I kept for over nine years. Many changes occurred over that period: marriage, divorce, my first major move out of town, and the death of my nineteen-year-old brother while he was driving under the influence.

My first encounter with coke was through one of my husband's friends, who stopped by our house one day and laid out eight hefty lines on the kitchen table. My drug of choice at that time was speed. Compared to the smaller-proportioned lines of crank I had experienced, these lines looked

ENORMOUS. I had never tried cocaine; I considered it to be a "hard" drug, in the same class with heroin and morphine. Never mind that I had popped nearly every kind of pill that existed. In my opinion, only junkies messed with hard drugs. As our friend whipped out a straw and quickly inhaled four of those gargantuan white streaks, I distinctly remember experiencing a feeling of shocked horror. Here was someone I knew pretty well, about to overdose in my kitchen! He handed me the straw next and said, "Go ahead, there are two for each of you."

My only previous experience with snorting white powder was crank. I knew that a line about one-tenth the size these were would keep me up for 24 hours or more. So there was no way I was going to ingest two of these heaps in their entirety. I took the straw and snorted up about half of one of the lines. My husband did the other half. Our friend quite happily polished off the remaining three. I kept watching him to see what it was going to do to him, at the same time waiting expectantly for the drug to take hold of me. Both areas were a big letdown. He never acted any differently, and I felt nothing. When he told us how much he paid for the stuff, I nearly fell over. "What a waste of money!" I thought. "I'll just stick to my speed, thanks!"

After my husband and I divorced, I moved to a small town a few hours' drive away. Weighing 80 pounds, I decided it was time to quit the speed, which I promptly replaced with alcohol. I was young and newly single and the bar scene appealed to me immensely. My ex was soon part of a "jet-setting" crowd: life in the fast lane, big cars, loose women, and lots of cocaine.

For about one and one-half years after the divorce, he came to visit me for the weekend, once or twice a month. He invariably brought along large quantities of coke and all sorts of paraphernalia. While I'm quite sure he was hoping to lure me back to him, I was equally aware that the only reason I allowed these visits was because I wanted to do his drugs. By this time I'd had enough exposure to cocaine to appreciate its finer qualities. These weekend binges fed my habit nicely. All I had to do was put out a little sex to a guy I'd been sleeping with for five years anyway. It seemed like a fine arrangement to me.

When I moved 3,000 miles across the country, I honestly believed it was because of job burn-out and my desire for a career change. What I can see now, is that I was pulling a classic "geographic."

I spent the next four years in a constant state of partying. Most of the coke was provided without charge. It wasn't long, however, before the neighborhood dealer was getting early morning calls from me for the quarter or half that I needed to get me through work that day, after a long, sleepless night of drinking and using.

The scenario changed quite a bit when I ran into an old high school buddy of mine from back East. We fell in love immediately and got married one and one-half years later. Our tastes in drugs were nearly identical: plenty of pot, a bottle of gin, and enough coke to keep us up all weekend.

We managed pretty well for a while, but soon the debts started building up. The parties were now extending on either side of the weekend. I could see we were getting into trouble, but I still believed we could turn it around if we only worked a little harder and cut back on the coke. After an extended period of unemployment, my husband and I began working. In my mind, we were all set up to turn things around for the better.

Instead, we got hooked on the pipe. I didn't want anything to do with the pipe, myself. Frankly, smoking it scared me to death. One night, however, I was sitting in the bedroom watching television while my husband and a couple of his friends were in the kitchen passing the pipe. I don't know if it was because it was the only drug in the house or if I just felt like I was missing out, but I suddenly walked into the kitchen and demanded a hit. "Where's mine?" were my exact words. This action came totally without any conscious decision on my part.

The guys were only too happy to load me up a rock. With that first hit, in the tiny instant it took me to burn it, I became a rock hound. I saw a television show once in which they interviewed a crack addict. When they asked him how long it took him to become addicted, he replied, "One hit, man, one hit." I knew *exactly* what he meant.

At first, we didn't use every day, but it seemed to get to that stage very, very quickly. I started living from hit to hit. Hitting the pipe was the first thing I did when I got home at night, and the last thing I did before I left for work in the morning. How I held on to my job is a total mystery. There were quite a few days when I just couldn't make it. More frequently, I'd go in blasted out of my mind. All day, I'd think, "Tonight I'm going to sleep," but by the time I headed out the door at 5:00 P.M., I was already obsessing on that hit I'd have waiting for me at home. Sometimes I'd be up for three or four days at a time, then go into a blackout crash, almost what you'd call a comatose state. When I woke up, it would start all over.

I felt as if I were living a dual existence: executive secretary by day, plodding through my work on autopilot; crazed crack addict by night, scamming money however I could to buy that one more rock. I was in total denial — nice girls like me didn't live like I was living. Yet, every so often, I'd get a moment of clarity and sheer terror would fill me, as I realized what my life had become. Then I would blame my husband, even though it was *me* demanding that he go out and score that one more twenty-dollar piece.

Every source of cash we had was gone; we'd borrowed from

every relative, the credit had exceeded its max, and the rent was two months overdue. I bailed out. I moved in with a friend of mine from work. She knew I was having problems at home, but thought it was just marital trouble. No one but my husband had any idea what was really going on at home. After three weeks of staying with my friend, I was able to pull together enough money to get my own place. I was so sure things would turn around now that I was away from that environment. Funny thing about addiction, though — once you've got it, it follows you wherever you go.

Within a week after I had moved into my new place, I agreed to let my husband join me. Within a matter of days, we were right back into the same routine. I felt like a trapped rat; there was nowhere left to go, and I was paralyzed with fear.

One night, while my husband was out on a drug run and I was plunged into a deep depression, a memory suddenly clicked in the back of my mind. I remembered a pamphlet I had found at work for something called the Employee Assistance Program. I had scanned it furtively at the time, glancing over my shoulder to be sure no one was watching me (after all, I didn't have a problem and I certainly didn't want anyone thinking that I did). A little voice in my head had prompted me to stash that piece of literature deep inside my desk for future reference, not that I would ever need it.

Sitting alone in our apartment, I felt utterly hopeless. I hated what my life had become. I was beginning to realize that I was not going to be able to change it on my own. The tears started falling uncontrollably. Through my stoned stupor, I vowed to call the number in that pamphlet the very next day.

Something, which I now know was my Higher Power, allowed me to fulfill that vow when I got to work the following day. I went to see one of the E.A.P. counselors. She referred me to an outpatient drug and alcohol treatment facility. I canceled my first appointment with them, but a week and a half later, I found myself in the enrollment office. I hadn't slept in three days. When they told me they wanted me to start that very night, I tried to protest, but somehow I knew it was time. The party was over.

I was introduced to recovery through the center. They immediately insisted I get involved in one of the Twelve Step programs. They told me it would be my consistent interaction with the fellowship of others in recovery that would keep me clean and sober. Though I went to meetings of various Twelve Step programs, it was in the rooms of Cocaine Anonymous that I really felt in tune with what was being said. I learned about the disease and came to find out that thousands of others have been able to rediscover themselves in a drug-free life, simply by following a few simple suggestions. The warmth and love I found filled me with a deep sense of happiness. I knew immediately that this was where I belonged.

A month after I got into the Program, my husband joined me. I'd love to be able to say we've been clean and sober ever since, but that is not the case. After a couple of months, we relapsed together at an office Christmas party. What started out as one drink, became a two-day coke binge. This stretched into six long weeks of using and drinking with renewed vigor. They say that it takes what it takes to get each of us to this Program. I believe my relapse was necessary for me, to reaffirm that getting high was not where I wanted to be. I had been told that after a period of abstinence, you pick up right where you left off in terms of your using/drinking habits. I'm here to tell you that, at least in my case, this was absolutely true.

When I take a look at how I got here and why I went back out, I believe I relapsed because I came in with underlying motives: I wanted to save the job and the marriage. After my relapse, neither of those things seemed nearly so important.

When I came crawling back, it was because I knew that if I didn't stop, I would die — plain and simple. The members of C.A. welcomed me home with hugs and understanding. Sobriety became my number one priority. I've been able to stay clean and sober ever since.

It took my husband a little longer to get back than me. Those were not easy times. We must have separated on at least four different occasions. But with the help of my Higher Power, my sponsor, and many, many friends in the Program, I made it through those difficult times. Today, we are both clean and sober and happier than we ever believed possible. We stay active in the Program, attend lots of meetings, and take on commitments whenever possible. It's become a way of life for us — one that we don't ever want to give up.

I always thought I had a pretty good life. Now, I know there is more to it than the selfish, materialistic point of view I used to hold. Because of this Program, I have been blessed with an "attitude of gratitude." I thank God on a daily basis for leading me here. By working the Twelve Steps in my life, not only can I keep this gift of sobriety, but I can also strive to be the best person I can possibly be. Cocaine Anonymous helped show me that this is not just a program of staying straight, it's a program of living and enjoying life to the utmost of our ability.

Addicted to crack cocaine? I thought it couldn't ever happen to a nice girl like me. But it did. If I could go back in time, I wouldn't change a thing, because it opened my eyes to an inconceivable level of existence and a realm of unlimited opportunity for happiness. It's available to me as long as I stay clean and sober, one day at a time.

8

TO BE THE BEST

As a teenager, he thought he had found everything he ever wanted in chemicals...until he found what he was really seeking...in recovery.

*T*REMEMBER, as I was growing up, that all I ever wanted was to be the best at something. I always thought of myself as just being average. Because I was so usual, I never felt like I fit in with everyone else. I figured if I were the best at any one thing, I would be accepted by my peers, and then I would be okay.

At first I tried sports; I could run but I wasn't the fastest. So I tried doing well in school, but my scores were not the highest. I tried to be popular, but I was too insecure to reach out.

One day, my big break happened; I found drugs. I was twelve years old. None of my friends could say they did that! Finally I had my claim to fame. My brother had some pot, and we smoked it. I coughed a lot and felt exhilarated because this was illegal. I then made sure that all of my friends knew that I was someone special. Surprisingly enough, my friends were not impressed. This was a disappointment. I did know the solution though: find new friends! This was easy enough. My new friends were really impressed with my drug use.

As time went on, the solution changed. Actually, I didn't need friends to be accepted. I suddenly realized that the drugs provided me with all the acceptance I needed. I had a new "best friend." Drugs and I did everything together. Having drugs with me made everything more fun. How could something that did so much for me be considered harmful? With this belief, the curse returned. In time, everyone I knew did drugs. I was no longer unique because I did drugs. I now had to be the best at using.

My father was a doctor and a using addict. I had access to the drugs that would make me king. I tried all combinations. The time between highs became less, the time spent high became longer, and the highs became higher. The only times I could remember feeling a sense of accomplishment were all drug-related.

Then the magic really happened. I was introduced to my best, best friend, my mentor, my wife. I was introduced to cocaine, and I took my love affair with drugs a step further. I was really committed. I spent no time sober. Every other aspect of my life was not as important: school, friends, work, dating, family. None of these mattered as much as the high. I went to school a few times a week so I could say I was in school. I had a girlfriend; not because I loved her, but because I was supposed to have one. Everyone could see my failing but me. Had you asked me at the time if something was wrong, I would have replied that things were never better. It was this way to the end. I was the walking dead and never knew it.

What happened next was that my father, in his disease, was placed into treatment. As he addressed his addiction, he realized that his children were also chemically dependent. I was soon to follow him into treatment. I was shocked at first that anyone could even think that my drug use was suspect. Quite against my will, I was admitted to an adolescent drug and alcohol program. I was seventeen years old. My status as the "best user" was challenged. My stories of drugs and conquest were not as good as the other patients' stories. On the other hand, I had to make it seem like I was only using socially so that these people would let me go home. The lies became too numerous to keep track of. I even tried to keep notes to remember what I told to whom. I was unsuccessful. I was caught and confronted.

The lies weren't working, so I decided to try this honesty thing. I was average again and depressed. People at the treatment center and at meetings tried to tell me that they could relate, but that only made things worse.

I kept a journal while I was a patient that I didn't share with anyone. Looking back in that journal I saw a pattern. At first, the denial started to slip. I went from having no problem, to maybe needing to cut down a little, to needing to cut down a lot, to being an alcoholic/addict. This process took about three months. In the end, I completed Step One.

Then came the God concept. As soon as I saw the term "Higher Power" followed by "God," I knew what was coming. I was a devout atheist and proud of it. Nobody was going to convince me otherwise. However, one counselor saw this as a challenge. He never told me to believe in God. He just told me to be open-minded. He argued for the existence of a kind and loving Higher Power, while I denied the possibility of an almighty Supreme Being that punished without reason. I argued for reason and science, while he explained with reason and science. The only reason I never admitted to accepting the possibility of a Higher Power to him was the little pride I had left. I really wasn't sure about the "God thing" so I used the Twelve Step group as a surrogate. Because it says that we "Came to believe," and not "We all of a sudden knew for sure," I had completed Step Two.

Then came the big one: turning my will and life over. I honestly didn't know what my "will" was or what it meant. I also had enough ego left to prevent me from asking anyone who might know. I *did* know what my life was, and it wasn't going to be turned over to anyone or anything. While I beat myself up over this for a few weeks, I noticed that many of my peers seemed to have no problem with understanding or practicing this. I finally broke down and asked one of the other patients how to turn my will and life over. I chose to ask the stupidest person I could find. We sat down. He asked if I wanted to turn my will and my life over. I said yes. He said I was done. Like a ton of bricks it hit me. All I had to do was make the decision. I had worked Step Three.

Steps One through Three took a total of about six months. This was also the amount of time I was in the treatment program. An amazing thing had happened over this time span. My last words to my using buddies when I knew I was going into treatment were, "If I come back from this trip sober, make me use until I beg for it." On the night before my discharge, I saw someone pick up an eleven-year token. I made a commitment to myself that I would be one of those people who stayed sober under any circumstances.

I returned home. At the first meeting I went to, I heard a speaker who really impressed me. I asked him for his phone number, and he became my sponsor. We reviewed Steps One, Two, and Three. I was told to take blank paper and pencil and start writing. My Fourth Step was 40 pages on regular notebook paper. I was so scared that, if Step Four said to be thorough, I was going to be meticulous. My sponsor read through my inventory and said, "That's it." I was very disappointed. I had heard horror stories about people's Fifth Steps. Mine went smoothly. I had expected pain and suffering.

By defining "shortcomings" and "character defects" I gained an understanding of the meanings of Steps Six and Seven. I could then see my character defects and my shortcomings and I was willing to make the effort to change.

Something else was happening about this time. I was at a point where I was getting on my knees to pray in the morning and at night, just to be open-minded. I never saw the burning bush. The room did not fill with light. I did not have this amazing awareness of God. I was, however, very humble. I was able to carry this humility into other areas of my life.

This was extremely helpful once I started the list of people I had harmed. After the list was complete, I contemplated the willingness to make these amends. I decided that willingness to make them all would not apply to me, because three of the people had moved out of state. I had no way of finding them or contacting them. As I laughed about this fact to myself, two of them called me. If I was still borderline about my faith in a Higher Power, that ended it. I had worked Step Eight and had already started on Step Nine.

I would like to say at this point that I made all of my amends and it was easy, but that's not quite how it went. Although I had the willingness, I still lacked some desire. It was difficult for me to say that I was sorry to all of these people while I still thought they first owed me some amends. It became a lot easier when I heard someone at a meeting say that making amends was saying that you were wrong, not that you were sorry. If you were sorry, then by all means say so, but don't say you're sorry if that's not how you feel. The point was to clean my side of the street, because I'm the one who is trying to stay sober.

After I finished making all of the amends on my list, I called my sponsor. We talked about Steps One through Nine. We decided that Steps Ten, Eleven, and Twelve would be my program for recovery on a daily basis.

This occurred at about the time I took my one-year token. I was really excited about celebrating my year. I kept thinking to myself, "One year! That's an impressive amount of time!" This thinking lasted until the end of my first year. I picked up my token, and remember being disappointed. One year was not that impressive any more. After all, if I had done it, so could anyone. I was back to being average. However, two years would be an accomplishment. That made sense to me!

During my second year I worked all Twelve Steps again, much like the first time. The second time through was a lot easier. I was going to about four to six meetings a week, and was comfortable at that level. My second year came and went like the first one. I have found this pattern to be true for all of my birthdays. I get really excited about my upcoming anniversary right up to that day, then I start to think. Without fail, the next year always seems like more of an accomplishment than the one I currently have.

At the time of this writing, I have nine years of sobriety and am 26 years old (Ten years...yeah, that seems like a lot!). I think that I have accomplished much. My plan for life while I was using was to use until I ran out of money and then kill myself. In sobriety, I have completed my B.S. degree at a university that I thought I could never get into. I even plan to go back for more. I have a job that I love; not because I make lots of money (I don't), but because I am comfortable with myself and who I am. This is true in all areas of my life because of this Program. I stick to the basics: Steps, meetings, sponsor.

Because I am willing to work this Program, I have been able to be the best at one thing, better than anyone else can ever be. I have found that I am the best at being me.

9

IN SICKNESS AND IN HEALTH

They found that couples can indeed make it in recovery.

*M*Y HUSBAND AND I are both recovering cocaine addicts. By the grace of God and with
the program of Cocaine Anonymous, each of us
has remained free from all mind-altering substances for over
three years. Today our lives are miracles, but there was a time
when neither of us would have believed recovery was possible.

I grew up in a family in which I was the youngest of three
girls. Though my parents never took drugs or drank exces-
sively, there were a lot of problems with the way they parented
their children. My father was overly critical, controlling, and
often verbally abusive. In contrast, my mother chose to avoid
conflict by standing behind my father's actions and being
silent whenever possible. In defending him, she became
emotionally unavailable to us.

During my school years I expended a lot of energy trying
to earn my father's approval. I applied myself to my studies,
volunteered at the hospital, performed community service,
made the basketball team, involved myself in the church, and
tried hard to be the perfect daughter. I learned pretty quickly
that I was far from perfect. I concluded that I was a defective
human being and that I was never going to be good enough,
pretty enough, or smart enough to earn the attention and
praise that I craved from my parents. At the age of twelve, I
finally gave up trying.

Throughout junior high and high school I rebelled in every
way I could think of. I ditched classes, hung out with the
"cool" crowd, snuck out at night, dated older men, and
discovered the thrill of being daring and "bad." I was intro-

duced to pot and alcohol. I began to experiment with as many other drugs as I could lay my hands on. I found acceptance among my drug-using buddies. I felt a part of a group for the first time. I liked myself more and felt my inhibitions slipping away whenever I was high.

Though my husband was the youngest of five children, he was raised as an only child because his brothers and sisters were so much older than he. His background is very similar to mine; even though there were no drug or alcohol problems in his household, his home life was dysfunctional, at best. As a teenager, he discovered that drugs and alcohol were the key to fitting in with his friends at school. Soon partying became the focus of his social life.

When we met on a blind date, I fell head over heels in love with him. We had the same values, the same type of upbringing, the same interests, and many friends in common. I knew without a doubt that he was the man I would someday marry. We began slowly, by dating for almost a year before living together.

We were at a party one weekend when a friend of ours showed us how to freebase cocaine. Cocaine is such a cunning, baffling, and powerful drug, that another full year went by without it giving us even a hint of a problem. We thought it was just a social drug; we only partied on the weekends, and we thought that we could quit any time we wanted.

We married two years after we met. Our drug use soon escalated. The next year passed by in a blur for both of us. We never stopped loving each other, but somehow our relationship began to fade in the shadow of our obsession to get and use cocaine. It was no longer a social drug. We stuck around the party only long enough to score coke. We then drove home, cooked it up, and smoked it. Some nights we went out three or four times on drug runs. We became paranoid whenever a car would pass by outside. We began to hide in closets. We fought horribly about the finances, who had to make a drug run this time, and who was smoking more than the other. When we fought, my husband would escape by going to bed. I would stay up scraping the pipe one last time or crawling around the floor for hours looking for rocks of cocaine that might have dropped. When we "came to" the following morning, utter despair and shame would prevent us from wanting to open our eyes.

By this time we knew, without a doubt, that we were addicted to cocaine. We could see our lives unraveling at the seams. We felt completely powerless to stop this from happening. At work we were performing badly and were often absent. We had high interest loans and no ability to pay them. We both had chronic coughs and other medical problems that we were too frightened to seek help for. Our parents were so concerned about our behavior that they stopped loaning us money once they realized we were being dishonest with them. We chose cocaine over jobs, food, health, and family, and came close to losing it all.

When I thought about getting help all I could come up with were excuses: my insurance wouldn't cover it, my parents would disown me, my husband would leave me, I wasn't that sick, I was much too hopeless. My sick mind came up with one other option, but even though I was tired of living, I was much too chicken to die. Many times I tried to find the courage to throw myself in front of a car as I walked along the highway near home.

By now we were so out of touch with reality and so far apart emotionally, that I never even considered my husband's desperation. Unbeknownst to me, he had tried to commit suicide one night by overdosing on cocaine and was angry to find himself still alive the next morning. We both felt hopeless, discouraged, and completely without options. Today I thank God for choosing the moment that He did to intervene in our lives.

It all ended when my husband drove over to his parents' house to borrow a vacuum cleaner. The next thing I knew, he was sobbing on the other end of the telephone. "What's wrong?" I asked. He said, "I told them!" "You told them what???" I asked. "I told them everything," he said. With mounting panic, I said, "YOU TOLD THEM WHAT???" He sobbed out, "I told them that I'm smoking cocaine, and I'm afraid I'm going to die!" At that point, he told me that his parents were going to drive him to a treatment center. He asked if would I like to go with him. I was so angry at him for betraying me and telling our deep, dark secret that I wanted to scream at him. What I ended up spitting out was, "Yes, I'll go with you. But if you think I'm going to break down and cry, you have another thing coming!" The counselor at the treatment center took one look at my angry, defiant face and zeroed right in on my husband. He stayed; I went home.

My parents admitted me for outpatient treatment about two weeks later. Those first few weeks were spent asking my family for support, paying off drug dealers, saying goodbye to our using friends, and trying to act as though my life wasn't falling apart when I went to work every day. In the first few weeks of treatment, I was too angry to get honest. When I did get honest about my drug use, I began to see that I had to work on my own life. I had to recover for me; not for my husband, not for my parents, not for his parents — but for myself. The day I accepted that I was a cocaine addict and that I was powerless over cocaine, was the day God began to work a miracle in my life.

In early recovery we did what was suggested. We attended 90 meetings in 90 days. We each found a sponsor. We used phone numbers, read the Big Book, and involved ourselves in service work. I sought out a Higher Power that could work in my life. My husband found a Higher Power that would work for him. I remember smoking a ton of cigarettes and going out for coffee after every meeting. How amazed I was to look around and realize that we had a whole new set of friends! Most importantly, neither of us took drugs; one day at a time, one hour at a time, sometimes one minute at a time.

We began again as if we were strangers. We didn't even know if we still liked each other, so we had to start out as if we were dating once again. We had to learn how to communicate with each other without working each other's programs, how to enjoy sex without drugs, and how to fight fairly. We even tried to time the roller coaster ride so that we both wouldn't crash and burn at the same time. We attended some meetings separately, because it was important for us to have time apart from each other, to air out fears, frustrations, and anger. We also attended a couples meeting where we could work through some of those problems together. We learned about codependency, and worked very hard to form an interdependent relationship instead. Now I have a night out with the girls, he has a boys' night out, and we reserve time for a "date night." We were told it was difficult for couples to make it in recovery, so we worked twice as hard to give our marriage the chance it deserved.

Marriages take continual effort on both parts. Ours is no exception. I'm sure there will always be days when we can't see eye-to-eye, and times when we don't like each other. But these moments pass quickly when we both take responsibility for our own actions and become willing to work on solutions and compromises *together*.

Today we know that Cocaine Anonymous works in our lives. The rage and anger we once felt is gone from our marriage. Our commitment to God, to each other, and to the Program continues to grow daily. We believe that God spared our lives for a purpose, and that he has a perfect plan for us. The Big Book gives us wonderful Promises to look forward to, and a vision of what life can be like if we work a program of recovery. Today those Promises are beginning to come true in our lives.

When I was using drugs, I knew I wasn't capable of being a parent. This caused me a great deal of sorrow. In sobriety, my husband and I were blessed with the birth of our first child, whose life is truly a miracle of this Program. Her chances of good health and happiness with two actively addicted parents would have been nonexistent three years ago. Thanks to Cocaine Anonymous she was conceived and carried into this world drug-free. She is everything we've ever dreamed of, and much more. I thank God for her daily.

We continue to attend meetings regularly, work the Steps, and involve ourselves in service work because these things help us to stay clean, one day at a time. If you are a newcomer in Cocaine Anonymous, or a committed couple in early recovery — take heart! You don't have to be in pain forever if you go to meetings, read the Big Book, work the Steps, and seek God. For those of you involved in a marriage or serious relationship: work hard to rebuild the communication and friendship that you've lost and, most importantly, give your relationship the time it takes to heal. Recovery from the disease of addiction is all about being happy, joyous, and free. The Program really does work — if you work it!

10

THE START OF A NEW LIFE
She now feels comfortable being a woman rather than one of the boys.

WHEN I WAS growing up, I was a true follower. I needed to be loved and I needed the approval of my peers. I thought very little of myself and depended on others to make me feel good inside.

I was raised in a small town of less than 1,000 people. Since both of my parents worked, my sisters, my brother, and I were raised by the help. Life was relatively normal until my father became an international executive and we were transferred overseas. It was quite a shock, going from a small town to a large, foreign city.

While living there, I was sexually abused by a man who worked for the family. He began molesting me when I was ten years old, and continued to do so for about a year. Even though I was frightened, I did not tell anyone. I felt that somehow I was responsible for his behavior, that it was my fault he was abusing me. I kept this a secret until I was twenty years old and quite drunk. As I look back, I can see that I used alcohol to help tell my deep, dark secret.

After three years abroad, my parents divorced. I began to drink. I also learned that attention from males helped me feel better about myself. Having a boyfriend made me feel like a "whole person." I preferred older men. In retrospect, I believe I was looking for a father figure.

I became a flirt; it was the only way that I knew how to communicate. I felt lost if I did not have a man around. Needless to say, the girls didn't like me. It was the start of my bonding with men and looking at women as enemies and rivals.

I moved a lot, but no matter where I was, I found drugs. I used cocaine for the first time in 1973. When I fell in love with cocaine, I *really* fell in love with it — the world looked beautiful; I knew all the answers; I was in control; I was euphoric. I loved the lifestyle of staying up late and going out all the time. I went out with men who could support me and my cocaine habit. I never ended a relationship with a man unless I had another man lined up. I did this so that I would never have to be alone; being alone terrified me. I didn't like who I was and went to any length not to look at myself. Being straight, without drugs or alcohol in my system, also terrified me, so I made sure that I was always high on something. Looking back, I am amazed I was so afraid. When I first got sober, the feeling of waking up with a clean and clear mind was the best experience I had ever had; certainly better than any high on drugs. What a waste of so many years!

I tried going to college, but found that I could not concentrate. I thought something was wrong with me. I did not realize that, because I was using so much cocaine by this time, my thought processes had been affected. Strangely enough, I had no problem thinking about my next line of cocaine.

My disease was getting progressively worse and worse. I only associated with people who used as much cocaine as I did. That way, I knew that nobody would tell me that I was using too much cocaine; that my life was getting way out-of-hand. I was disoriented most of the time. I had hallucinations and heard voices. I was paranoid; I thought that all telephones, even the public ones on the streets, were tapped. My friends all carried guns and dealt cocaine. I thought invisible bugs were on my body and I consulted several doctors to determine the cause. I coughed up blood.

I went to a free clinic because I knew that it would be safe to tell them that I was using cocaine. The doctors there told me that I had to stop using in order to stop coughing up blood.

I thought about it and realized that giving up cocaine wasn't even an option. I then became so paranoid that I couldn't leave my house. I finally felt so desperate that I overdosed on some pills. I was hospitalized and released, but I did not stop using alcohol and drugs.

I was careless about where I went and who I talked to. I was beaten and almost raped. I did not think that my cocaine and drug use was related to these events.

By that time, I had no place to go. I had no friends and no money. I called my mother, an alcoholic who had stopped drinking a few years before. She took me to a detoxification center. I was 25 years old. That was the last day I used cocaine.

Asking for help was the start of a new life. I became educated about addiction. I learned that cocaine use was the cause of my problems, not the cure for them. As time went on, I began to realize that alcohol was also part of my problem. I attended some Twelve Step meetings but found that I did not feel comfortable talking about my cocaine addiction in them.

Cocaine Anonymous had not yet been founded, so I went to some other Twelve Step fellowships. I could not identify with the street aspect of drug use. Again I felt I had to hide my own addiction and what it was like for me. I felt, without realizing it, that I was terminally "unique." I knew I had to do something so that I would not start using cocaine again.

My best friend and I decided to start a Cocaine Anonymous meeting. We got together with two other recovering addicts, and although a lot of people were against it, saying there was no need for another Twelve Step fellowship, we went ahead with it anyway. We met week after week, just the four of us. Gradually, the idea took hold, and more and more people started coming to the meeting. Though we had many growing pains in the beginning (not that we still don't today), our Fellowship kept growing and growing.

It's hard for me to talk about God, but I need to say that God is a part of my life today. Without my faith and God's guidance, none of my sober life would have been possible. God, as I understand Him, is kind, loving, and accepting. God's will is what's best for me. As I sit here writing this, it is my tenth sober anniversary (birthday). I am so grateful for the miracle of my sobriety that words cannot describe the way I feel.

The best gift I have been given is that I like myself. The emptiness, the void, in my stomach is gone. Drugs, alcohol, food, and men couldn't fill it. Sobriety, the ability to look in the mirror and like who I see, and God filled the void. I learned that it can't be filled from the outside; it has to come from within.

The hardest issues for me have been the "female" ones. I didn't realize how much cocaine use affected me as a woman. I used cocaine and other drugs to numb my feelings of being sexually abused. I used cocaine and other drugs in order to be with men. I was promiscuous; it was the only way I knew how to act. I thought that promiscuity would get me the love I needed. I knew that promiscuity would get me the drugs I wanted. My drugging helped me deny that I had an eating disorder. When I had P.M.S., without realizing it, I used drugs and alcohol to cover up the symptoms. I disliked other women; they were the enemy.

Today I have overcome all of these issues. I feel comfortable being a woman, not "one of the boys." I didn't used to know what I wanted to be when I grew up, but today I am happy to say that I do. When I grow up, I want to be a sober female member of Cocaine Anonymous. Thank you, Cocaine Anonymous for giving me back my life.

11

FIRE IN MY BRAIN

He never thought that he could quit cocaine on his own. When he surrendered to a Higher Power, the Twelve Steps and the Fellowship of Cocaine Anonymous did the rest.

*F*OR THE PAST seventeen years, I have faithfully written and maintained a daily diary. It is from these entries that I recount my story, drawing from them my life experiences and the insanity of those years.

My first experience with cocaine was at a private party in the early seventies. I was so strung out on downers and alcohol that I could not even tell which drug was affecting me. It was several years before I tried cocaine again.

Over the years, I witnessed several acquaintances being arrested for dealing cocaine. The end result was the forfeiture of all their possessions, not to mention having to do hard time in state prisons. I swore not to get involved with cocaine.

My thinking and my actions changed when I moved, in the late seventies, as a result of a job transfer. Since my live-in girlfriend chose not to relocate with me, I was lovesick. Somewhere I had read that celebrities had used cocaine as a substitute to ease the pain of lost love relationships. Why not me? I found a connection and was soon using cocaine to lift my spirits.

At this time in my life, I stopped drinking alcohol and started attending a Twelve Step fellowship. I did not take another drink of alcohol for the next four years. However, I began to increase the number of times I snorted cocaine. I began to read more and more about this "White Lady" with which I was becoming infatuated. She possessed powers that I could identify with and that I wanted. I read about how to wash and clean out my nose, what vitamins to take, and what herbs to use to detox. I also read claims about how this drug was not addictive. This "nonaddictive drug" told me what I wanted to hear and promised to share with me some of her secret powers.

I was sharing a house in the mountains with two female housemates, one of whom was a drug dealer. I had a new job that required extensive out-of-state traveling. My arrangement with my drug-dealing housemate was this: I would wire her money and she, in turn, would "overnight" me a weekend's supply of cocaine.

The turning point in my life, when cocaine use became an obsession, was in May of 1980, during a stop to gamble in Nevada when I won over $1500. I called home to share my good luck with my two housemates. They assured me that there was a shipment of cocaine coming in that night, and that they would leave a gram for me in my dresser drawer.

Instead of staying and gambling more, I suddenly decided to drive nonstop to my house in the mountains where my reward would be waiting. I drove fast and hard for the next nine hours, with my mind focused on the gram of cocaine awaiting my arrival. Finally, I arrived. I found the house dark. My housemates had split and left a note in my dresser drawer: "Sorry, we used yours up and will replace it tomorrow." Needless to say, I was outraged. The next day I purchased a large amount of cocaine from another connection. I swore to my date, "I will never ever be out of cocaine again." My next step was to rent a safe-deposit box. I placed sealed vials in it and replenished my inventory whenever possible. I was in control. Now, I always had a supply.

I continued to use and abuse cocaine. All the while, I kept my diary filled with my ongoing, day-to-day, life experiences. I even kept daily records of not only when I used cocaine but how much I spent for my ever-increasing habit. On

December 15, 1981, I wrote the following in my diary, entitled "Fire in my Brain":

"In two weeks of attempted self-destruction, I have spent $510 for 5.25 grams of instant pleasure. Instant pleasure — HA HA! An ongoing obsession — Addiction with a capital A — a never-ending HABIT. Yet, all actions, all desires and guilt to end this Madness have failed. Time after time and again and again — the need — the desire — the want — WINS. And the purchases add up, the craving is never satisfied — always the fear of no more or of running out. Yes, A FIRE IN MY BRAIN. An addiction with NO END BUT THE ULTIMATE END. In the meantime — day by day — the suffering from overdoing — the long, long nights of laying there cursing this HABIT — this addiction — only waiting to arise the next morning and begin again. The constant process of — Reasoning, the money — the priority of the money now and still no end. The process of priorities and the GRAM — the need now — the desire — the craving WINS — again and again. The first line is only the beginning — then followed quickly by the second and then the third and the fourth line and on and on. Just to feel the sensation of the uplift. But, wait — then the need — then the craving takes over — then comes the PRIORITY OF DO I HAVE ENOUGH? Do I have money for more? Always the answer is YES — THE PRIORITY WINS AGAIN. This FIRE IN MY BRAIN is now an addiction — an overwhelming, ongoing obsession with no reasonable or logical solution to end — to cease this FIRE IN MY BRAIN. My health? My self-esteem? My poor nose? My overall functions and feelings? No answers — just more vitamins and more guilt and I am again a loser to the need — the desire — the wants and the cravings... I continue to feed this endless fire — continue to place the priority of this addiction as the WINNER in my life. But, by this being the winner, "I" — the reality of ME is the ULTIMATE REAL LOSER. I hope and I pray for a SOLUTION to become a real winner and not a loser!"

The solution was still years away. I was involved in a love

relationship and used cocaine to control it. When the power of cocaine lost out and that relationship ended, I started drinking again. Over the next few years, I proceeded to mix alcohol, cocaine, and pharmaceuticals. At times, I would isolate for days on end. My circle of so-called friends consisted mainly of lowlife individuals and drug dealers.

I began a new love relationship and promised her that I would not use cocaine. Soon I was denying my usage when confronted. I was arrested for drinking and driving. Part of my sentence was that I had to attend drunk-driving school. I showed up for the hearing and sentencing wired and wasted on cocaine. I had promised myself when I had stopped drinking years earlier that I would never be abusive in a love relationship again. However, when my girlfriend canceled a date at the last minute, I verbally abused her over the phone and went on my last drunk.

I made a decision to try a Twelve Step program again. I was concerned about the fact that I had tried one before, only to quit alcohol and become addicted to cocaine. I knew that somehow, some way, I had to stop using cocaine. Because I could not say no in certain situations or to people who were still using, I forbade any cocaine in my residence.

Fifty days after my last drink, on a Saturday morning, the front door opened and there they were — four county narcotic agents, wearing bullet-proof vests. Two of them quickly placed guns to my head, while another read me my rights. The fourth agent showed me a warrant for my arrest, saying, "You know that it is finally all over with."

The narcotics agents were upset that they could not find any cocaine in the house. However, I was charged with possession of various pills and conspiracy to traffic. My own diary and my personal accounts of using and abusing cocaine were later used as evidence against me.

My problems increased: my girlfriend broke up with me; I

was presented a 30-day eviction notice; I was notified of an upcoming I.R.S. audit with a staggering balance due. I was told to hire the best lawyer I could find, which I did. He was not cheap. My youngest daughter was expelled from boarding school and her mother sent her to live with me. My expensive car blew its engine, leaving me with no transportation. In one week, I had gone from assets to liabilities. Impending doom had now set in.

I was too scared to use. Someone suggested that I attend other Twelve Step programs. In my area, at a drug treatment facility, a weekly meeting of Cocaine Anonymous had just started. I began to attend this meeting. I finally heard the message: that I could not take *anything*, no matter what. Over a period of 30 years of drinking and doing drugs, I had painted myself into many a corner and had learned how to paint myself out. I trusted no one and I was not going to change. I was just not going to drink, take a pill, or do a line of cocaine again.

Over the next 90 days, I attended as many C.A. meetings as I possibly could. I chaired a C.A. meeting when I had less than 90 days clean and sober. I was full of fear, anxiety, doubt, and negativity. To add to my burden, I had the fear of having to do hard time. However, I was too full of stubborn pride to give in and change my attitude, my thinking, or my actions. I only knew that I could not take *anything*, no matter what.

Finally, I had to deal with my brother, who was very religious, and my mother, who I didn't want to see or be with. I made excuses so that I would not have to deal with them. My brother finally confronted me about my excuses. I finally admitted to him that I was falling apart and that I was really scared. His reply was, "Have you ever tried praying?" My answer was "No, I haven't." All of a sudden, I found myself down on my knees on the kitchen floor. I started praying, and finally I surrendered. I remember saying, "God, please take me and help me. I am throwing in the towel. Whatever it takes, I am willing to do it. Please help me. I can't live this way any longer!" Since that day, I have never felt the compulsion, or had the obsession, to drink or use.

My next step was one of action. I went looking for, and soon found, a sponsor. He was what we call an old-timer. Doing the Third Step was extremely difficult for me. My sponsor kept telling me that if I thought that I had taken the Third Step, it didn't take. I finally saw the light and discovered that this is a spiritual program and that God, as I understand Him, is of my own choosing. God, to me, is a loving, caring, and forgiving Higher Power. I did not have to beat up on myself any longer. The Fourth and Fifth Steps freed me from the fog of my many self-inflicted and self-centered fears.

Because of my heavy involvement in Twelve Step meetings, my lawyer arranged plea bargaining and kept me from doing hard time. I was placed on heavy-duty probation and had to participate in state-ordered drug counseling so they could monitor me. I worked with my drug counselor on my Sixth and Seventh Steps. I shared my amends with my sponsor and with my counselor. In meetings, I often share my experience, strength, and hope, and how I work the Steps.

With the working of each Step, came emotional releases, personal growth, more tools to use and, finally, change. I now feel "a part of" instead of "apart from." I even had to put God on my amends list. In my seven-plus years of using cocaine I had forgotten about God and had shut Him out of my life; as cocaine had been my Higher Power. The "White Lady" lied to me all those years and all those endless times that I sought her power. I came to understand and believe that there is only one Power and that one Power is God. I was home — finally. I found a Fellowship that would love and accept me. I didn't have to prove myself any longer. Finally, I was a member. Finally, I'd found love and acceptance. Many of the Promises have been fulfilled as I have gone to great lengths to make my amends. I am now reunited with my entire family. I have cleared much of the wreckage of my past. Over the past seven years, the tools that I have now, the changes, the growth, and my new attitude toward life have continued to amaze me. I had to unlearn old habits, old thinking, and not only become willing and honest, but teachable. However, I did not do this alone. I now know a new Source of Power. I am now grateful for my new lease on life.

My day begins and ends with a simple prayer: "God, take me today and let me be who You want me to be. Let Thy will, not mine, be done. God, help me to NOT take a drink of alcohol or a mind-altering drug today. Amen." I show up each day and God does all the rest.

12

WHAT FINALLY HAPPENED...

He had plenty of chances, had been warned many times. What finally happened made the least amount of sense: he surrendered.

THROUGHOUT MY LIFE, I could have given you plenty of reasons why things were all screwed up. Today, I know that "the why is a lie!" It's taken a few years of recovery in Cocaine Anonymous and extensive inventory work to make the shift from being a victim of my parents, family, society, jobs, etc., to one of being fully responsible for all facets of my life. It's been a very simple process, one that began with acceptance of Step One in its entirety, after eight months of trying recovery on my terms.

I was born the eldest of five. I used to say that I didn't ask to be brought into this world. I never went without food, clothing, shelter, or education, yet I consistently had a large case of the "wants." Not once did I feel secure and satisfied with my life or those in it. There was no active addiction or alcoholism in my family, neither was there sharing of feelings nor much intimate interaction. I learned to be seen and not heard, to be tough, not to trust others, and to fear my parents and authority figures. When I was punished, many times it was physically. It seemed as though I was constantly in trouble. Deep within myself, I began to believe that I was bad and incapable of doing the "right" thing. My defects grew by leaps and bounds as I learned to hate the world and myself.

I remember a time when I was with a group of football players and my father. We were denied service in a restaurant because some of the men were black. After a great deal of discussion between my father and the proprietor, we were seated and served. I knew at that time how deeply my father cared for these men and all others, and yet I didn't believe that he loved me. I began a pattern of attempting to win his love through achievements. I wanted to be black. It seemed as though no matter how hard I tried, I was never good enough. Later, I discovered that I continued this pattern in all of my relationships. I expected approval, applause, or love. When I didn't receive it, I used this as an excuse to leave or to not be responsible. My payoff was to remain a victim, living constantly in self-pity. It was in Cocaine Anonymous that my first sponsor informed me that "sympathy was between shit and syphilis in the dictionary."

My first drink came when I was fourteen. I started smoking that same evening. From the beginning, I was never a person to moderate. That night was no exception; I drank half a quart of scotch. Looking back, I see where that drink saved my life; I found the release which was so necessary to get me beyond myself, my feelings of shame and anger, and my desire to die. That night there were no words negating my existence. Amazingly enough, 23 years later, the person I shared that quart with is also in recovery.

Life got good with drink. It got better with the addition of sex. All at once, I had the world by the tail, though later the tail turned out to belong to a 900-pound gorilla. It was at this point that I lost virtually all touch with the small amount of reality left in my life, a state which persisted until I found recovery eighteen years later.

My behavior deteriorated rapidly. As a result of never being home, poor grades, and extremely rebellious behavior, I began to receive more and more punishment. If life got good with drink and sex, it got even better when I discovered drugs, using five hits of speed at age sixteen. Again I found myself catapulted to a new height of life. It allowed me to do more and more and more. I felt as though I was above all laws, all morals, and all persons. Not once did I realize that I was the problem; I was convinced it was "them." Later, through cocaine psychosis, "them" came to life in the walls, the trees, and everywhere I looked. I was incapable of telling the truth even when I wanted to.

I became involved in the "good ol' boy" distribution network of illicit substances. I wore nicknames such as Animal, Mute, and Mr. Electric with pride. It wasn't until I came to Cocaine Anonymous that my real name meant anything to me, or I meant anything to myself.

After high school, I attended a military junior college where I played my last couple of years of football. It was clear to me that I was never going to be that fast. I wasn't interested in school or sports. After three semesters, actually two days before the end of my third semester, they drummed me out of the Corps of Cadets.

I was told by my father that I had 30 days to get a job and get out. This was a case where all was not lost, as that job was on an offshore oil rig. I have remained in that business to this day. Part of my denial was that I had never lost a job. It never occurred to me that the crazy people I worked around were a sign of my own questionable sanity. Today, one of the miracles of this Program is that I am now part-owner of a small company. This is a direct result of painstaking work, application of the Principles and the Twelve Traditions, and not doing cocaine, one day at a time.

I decided to marry. This marriage lasted nine years to the day. My wife stuck it out through one heart attack, one attempted suicide, and an overdose; as well as the lies, tears, and fears that go with being married to a full-blown maniac. While I wasn't prone to physical violence, I emotionally abused her and pushed her to the point of violence, as she continued to fill my need to be punished, a need that I arrived at the doors of C.A. with.

I had found cocaine before that marriage and had quit cocaine at the beginning of it. But cocaine soon reappeared in my life. I convinced my wife that it was the sensible thing to do. I also convinced her that it was a good product to distribute and that the clientele was upscale. For the next few years, my wife and I went to work, partied, fought, and made up, almost as a daily ritual. We would both go from wanting to get rid of the stuff to wanting to get more, within that same day.

I was roaring merrily through life; I felt invincible. But one day, while driving down the highway to a job, I overdosed and had a heart attack. Then, at age 32, I attempted to kill myself with cocaine. Today, both of these events show me the power of the God of my understanding and the existence of God in my life, even before I'd found my own faith.

By the time I arrived in treatment, I had overdosed three more times. I had lost my wife, all of my friends were afraid of me, and I lived each day full of terror. I couldn't breathe or sleep without cocaine. It took an eight ball at night to lay in bed. I wanted to bathe in it. No matter how much I had, it was never enough. I used it on all of my food and in my drinks. It took two and one-half years of recovery before I fully recovered from all of the visual and auditory hallucinations caused by my addiction.

My recovery was actually initiated by a psychiatrist who informed me that it was very apparent I wasn't afraid to die; rather, I was afraid to live life on life's terms. Somehow, I knew that he was telling the truth. This was the day I filed for divorce: six days after my most recent overdose and 286 days before I finally accepted Step One. You see, after treatment I intellectually understood the first half of Step One, and though I attended from 20 to 22 meetings a week, I relapsed on my 87th day. Why? Simply because I wasn't willing to give up my "friends" or dealing drugs. I didn't believe them when they said my friends didn't care. Hell, I knew they cared. They helped me get money and drugs. They had saved me on two occasions when I overdosed. They protected me. I didn't accept the love in the rooms of Cocaine Anonymous. I finally realized that my old buddies did care; they cared much the same as a pack of wild dogs do, for survival purposes only. We were incapable of anything more meaningful.

What finally happened... after entering the Program in 1986, I had six relapses. My time in sobriety got shorter and shorter, and my relapses more and more frequent. Each relapse represented failure to take action on my part. I never "slipped" on anything but a waxed floor or ice.

The first relapse was my last attempt at dealing cocaine and crank. It was for a party. As usual, I felt the need to bring the party to the party. This relapse lasted five weeks. The next one, after another six days sober, lasted a week. Again it was due to my inaction: I wouldn't drive to meetings. I was afraid because I didn't get to know anyone in the rooms. I wouldn't get a sponsor. I didn't quit associating with people who dealt or used.

My third relapse was after 47 days of sobriety and lasted for three horrible days. The auditory and visual hallucinations occurred with my first line of cocaine. I prayed to God, "PLEASE, I'VE GOT TO STOP — HELP ME!" I learned during this relapse that God would help, but that I needed to quit copping cocaine in order for God to help me stay away from it. Therefore, I needed to call my sponsor before I copped, not afterwards. I had never before called my sponsor until it was over. This was the last time I used cocaine.

The reasons for the next three relapses were simple: I wouldn't give up pot or my old buddies. I relapsed the last time because I didn't get honest about the fifth time.

They say we should remember our last high, and I do. I didn't get off. I didn't finish my first drink because, during that drink, the message of recovery and love that had been shared with me daily for almost a year shot through my soul. I left that bar on a Saturday night with a newfound freedom.

Finally, after my first sponsor told me to "please blow my #%*@ing brains out," I decided to try all of the suggestions. This was a month after my first C.A. meeting.

I accepted Step One as it relates to my addiction, my thinking, and my emotions. I came to believe in Step Two and began to drive 618 miles a week to attend three meetings. I made a decision in Step Three and followed it up with the necessary action in Steps Four through Nine. I began to feel and see the Promises materializing in my life, one day at a time.

When I began daily application of all the Principles, I tried to help the persons suffering. In my book, this included the person with ten years, as well as the newcomer; after all, none of us has more than a daily reprieve.

Each day, I am given the opportunity to witness the power and love of God manifested in several people's lives as they too are transformed from a state of hopelessness and despair, to joy and happiness.

I am grateful to C.A. for the literature piece "Who Is a Cocaine Addict," as I was one who 'couldn't breathe without cocaine.' I am grateful to God and to the Fellowship of Cocaine Anonymous for its unconditional love. Three and one-half years ago, someone told me that if I learned to live the Twelve Traditions in my life, I would never have a problem with another person. As a result of that conversation and my service work in this Fellowship, I have learned to live one day at a time in harmony with all people as members of my family. Today, when I choose to be, I am free, happy, and at peace. Presently, I am on an airline flight returning from a trip to make a living amends. I am a grateful recovering cocaine addict and a proud member of this beautiful Fellowship.

13

A PIPE DREAM
Everybody's caretaker; through recovery, she learned to take care of herself.

WAS BORN in the South. As fate would have it, I was born with a birth defect called a harelip. From the time my mother saw me, she hated me. How do I know this? She told me. For many years, from the age of two weeks to seventeen years, I was physically abused by my mother. Some of the abuse was beatings with fishing rods and electrical cords. One time, I can remember having my head shoved into a nail in the wall. Once she even shut a window down on my arms. That's just the tip of the iceberg.

My parents were bootleggers and introduced me to alcohol. At the age of fifteen, I was sexually abused by my mother and my stepfather. I started to drink to hide the resulting pain and shame that I felt. Though at the time I did not know it, my mother was an active alcoholic.

My natural father died when I was twelve years old. I loved him very much. I was very mentally unstable. I related love to sex and, needing stability, turned to older men for a father image. By living through these experiences, I grew up really fast.

By the age of fifteen, I'd become pregnant by a twenty-five-year-old man, at age seventeen by another man who was twenty-seven years old, and at age nineteen by one who was thirty years old. I thought that by having children, I would have someone to love me for me. I became very withdrawn. I tried religion of all types; I was looking for forgiveness. I blamed myself for this hell.

When I was sixteen, I met the man that I'm married to now.

He was married with eight kids. As fate would have it, I fell in love. This man became my idol, my knight in shining armor. After years of fooling around, we decided to live together. At least I was rescued from my mother.

When I was 21, my oldest sister drowned, leaving two young children. Eleven months later, my mother died of a heart attack. Three months before she died, she told me that she loved me. I told her that it really didn't matter anymore because I was grown. She left three other teenaged children as well as a twenty-year-old who was mentally retarded. It was left up to me to finish raising them because I was the oldest and no one else would take them. The two youngest of these were heavily into drug use. My younger sister had a child too, and was expecting another any day. So, by the age of 21, I had nine children to raise. By that time, I had started experimenting with downers, uppers, tranquilizers, antidepressants, beer, and cocaine. I found that I could cope if I was high on something. I tried marijuana, but couldn't handle the smoke.

I got married at the age of 26; my husband was 40. For about 11 years I had a good life. I wanted for nothing. I was an active member in the community and a youth counselor in the church I attended. I finished high school after being out of school for 20 years. I studied cosmetology and attended college for two and one-half years. I was there for my children all the time. I tried to give them everything I didn't have when I was growing up; always the best that money could buy. For once in my life, I was happy. I drank socially and tooted cocaine occasionally.

As fate would have it again, my husband, who suffered from asthma all his life, was diagnosed with emphysema. Despite all of the pain and suffering I had experienced, his illness affected me the most. I felt loss, hurt, anger, and fear; you name it. This man was my life, my all-and-all. What was I going to do? I started drinking more alcohol and tooting more cocaine to cope with my depression. As this was not enough, I turned to another man who was also an addict, though I didn't know it at the time. I was so in need of someone to care about me. For a while we had a good relationship. He didn't let me see him do anything with drugs except toot a little cocaine or smoke marijuana. I didn't feel comfortable in this relationship, but I was scared to let go. I did not want to be alone.

One day, he said he was going to show me how much he loved me. He was going to let me get high with him. He cared so much for me that he taught me how to smoke cocaine. First, he showed me how to cook it for him, then how to fire it up. I experimented for about two months, then I felt I didn't need his company anymore. I had finally found what I was looking for; something that would block out all of the hurt and pain that I was feeling. I was now living in a pipe dream. Sex no longer mattered. Crack cocaine became my husband, my best friend, and my lover because it gave me a feeling of peace. Nothing else in life really mattered.

It became an every-weekend thing, I spent all my money on it. In three months time, I had spent a very large sum of money but had never once smoked crack by myself. I became the joke of the rock house because I let everyone use me. I would spend hundreds of dollars on drugs in a night, then share it with everyone in the rock house. I could not stand for other addicts to fuss about not having cocaine. To keep peace and keep in my place, I would share.

This is an example of a day of my getting high: I would wake up depressed, if I got any sleep at all due to my husband's illness, get paid, or get money from my lawyer (I had a pending lawsuit). I didn't have to go to the drug dealer, all I had to do was send for him. He would bring me what I wanted. I would buy at least five eight balls in a day.

When my money ran out, I would find something to sell.

I went to old friends, relatives, and even my pastor to borrow money, using my husband's illness as an excuse. I stole checks and money from my daughter and my stepdaughter. I even stole my husband's S.S.I. checks. At one time, my insurance company sent me a check for a considerable amount. I spent it all in one night, in one rock house, on about six people. The next morning I couldn't even get a ride home. I took my lump sum income tax refund check to the drug dealer on a Saturday. By the following Monday I owed him more than half the check. By the time Tuesday came, I had spent the rest.

My money was getting short. Everybody was turning down my requests to borrow money. Since I was a big spender, drug dealers would front me cocaine. I continued to smoke crack cocaine for about eight months, still thinking that I did not have a problem. The stolen checks finally caught up with me, and I had to deal with my family. They all thought I was too strong to mess with drugs. Little did they know, I was only human.

I went to a 21-day treatment center, mainly to get away from everyone. While I was there, I faced my past. I talked about my abuse openly with my children, and with my husband, who had already known for years. I stayed there for the 21 days thinking that I would be all right as long as I didn't smoke any cocaine. I told myself I could still drink and toot cocaine; the smoking is what got me into trouble. I did all right for about six months. Little did I realize that my reason for turning to drugs in the first place was still there.

I was still isolated from everyone. My husband was in and out of the hospital where he was on life-support in the last stages of his illness. Sometimes, even the doctors would give up. This only made me feel worse. I kept feeling a part of me was slipping away. No one knows what this kind of hell feels like until he or she actually experiences it.

I went to Cocaine Anonymous meetings for about two

months and was in an aftercare program. I justified stopping that program because I was needed at home; I lied to myself. I never thought about working the Twelve Steps.

I needed help to stop crying, so I went back around some of my "old playgrounds and playmates." In a flash, I was right back in the scene, smoking crack cocaine. By this time, I had settled my lawsuit. I did manage to wait to start smoking until after I had spent the majority of my settlement replacing material things, buying a car, and trying to get back on my feet. After I had done all that, I told myself that it was time to get high. I deserved it because I had paid my dues. But I was wrong; I was right back in hell.

I had bought enough jewelry to cover my neck, and both hands and wrists two or three times. I immediately sold all of it to drug dealers. I pawned my car to someone I knew I wouldn't even give a ride to. I walked the streets at night begging for money and telling lies. I even broke into my own home and stole the air conditioner, pawned the microwave, and took money from my sick husband. I told lies to my youngest daughter to get money and jewelry from her to pawn. I even took the drug dealer to my home to tell my husband lies in order to get money.

I found myself in some of the worst places. I would be smoking in a rock house dressed up in a one-hundred-dollar dress. I found myself almost getting shot because some addict had stolen some cocaine from a dealer. After the dealer shot through the door, I vowed to stop getting high. How many addicts have said that?

One day I looked in the mirror and I saw myself. My hair was short and slick, my face was broken out, and my eyes were bloodshot. I was wearing a T-shirt and a pair of jeans. I saw the person I never wanted to become. I hated myself so much I wanted to die. I soaked my wool coat in gasoline. After wrapping my body in the coat, I struck a match. But something or someone, I know now that it was my Higher Power, saved me. I came to my senses and very quickly took the burning coat off. I was left without one single burn.

Finally, I prayed to God. I asked for God's forgiveness and the strength to help me overcome my problems with drugs. I had stopped praying before because I felt unworthy of God's love. I hated myself. Through prayer, I got an answer in my heart. I knew where it had come from.

I felt that I would not benefit from going back through a 21-day program. I knew that I had to first admit that I was an addict. I told myself, my husband, and my children. I called a counselor at the hospital. He said that I knew what I had to do. That day, I walked back into a C.A. meeting and admitted that I was an addict. I said I had relapsed, though I hadn't really, because I was never clean. I started going to meetings regularly.

At certain intervals of sobriety, each person receives a chip for 30 days, 60 days, and so on. It was truly an accomplishment when I received my first chip. I also reentered aftercare, went twice a week, and attended other Twelve Step programs.

I learned to work the Twelve Steps. This was, and continues to be, hard work. I no longer feel shame from the past or fear for the future. I have turned my life over to God's will. In the Fellowship of C.A. I have been given a feeling of unconditional love through coming together with other addicts to share our pain and experience of cocaine use and recovery.

Through recovery, I have learned that I no longer have to be a crutch for anyone, but that by holding hands, we can walk together. In my heart, I know recovery is a great change, a change in myself more than a change in people, places, or things. My life is now centered around my recovery. I must stay clean for myself, not because someone else wants me to. I attend at least eight meetings a week. I share my experience with other recovering addicts. I have daily meditation with my Higher Power, who is God. I no longer use any drugs. This includes alcohol because it, too, is a drug. I have learned to love myself.

I still face the problems of daily life, but I have now learned how to deal with them. If I cannot handle a problem, I just turn it over to God, and He handles it. Through recovery, I earned back the respect and trust of my family. Life gets better each day. God sends me a blessing every day because he keeps me clean and sober. I know that I can stay sober only one day at a time. I got the tools to stay clean and sober through C.A. It's up to me to use them. The meetings, the Twelve Steps and, most of all, my belief in a Higher Power have helped me to stay sober for 22 months.

Recovery works only if I work it. Most of all, I take one day at a time. Today I will work an honest program of recovery.

Remember, if someone doesn't tell you that they love you today, I do. I really mean it, because you are the me that I was, and you can soon be the me that I am today.

14

THE COURSE OF SOBRIETY

She went from a commitment to cocaine, to a commitment to recovery.

I HAD A bad day today. I was anxious, depressed, and angry. I just wanted it to end. On my way home from work, a huge white moon floated out from behind dark clouds. It made me smile — an almost too-perfect metaphor. In the bigger picture, in the face of that moon, it was hard to stay so wrapped up in my problems. There was once a time when the only way I could have coped with a day like this was to saturate myself with chemicals. There was also once a time when I couldn't hold a job, much less appreciate the sight of the moon.

My drug of choice was cocaine. I used anything and everything else, but cocaine was my favorite. I loved it with a passion that, in the end, nearly killed me. In the final years of my drug abuse, I was skeletal, paranoid, prone to cocaine-induced convulsions, and involved in an emotionally and physically abusive relationship. I was dead inside. I was numb, as if the cocaine had penetrated my very core. I didn't care about anything. Going into a rehab was more about just being too exhausted to continue my endless search for cocaine, than about wanting to get help.

It was in that hospital that I first heard about the Program, the Twelve Steps, and the possibility of a drug-free life. Although I subsequently relapsed several times after I left the hospital, some of what I learned there about my drug addiction stuck with me with a startling tenacity. It eventually took hold. I've been sober for over three years now; a fact which occasionally surprises me, as it once seemed impossible.

I started using drugs when I was fifteen years old. I was an especially insecure adolescent, which in itself is not particularly unique. I always felt different from my peers, as if I were branded somehow. The fact that my family moved around constantly from coast-to-coast, and then to Europe, did not help the sense of rootlessness that I felt. There was also the constant friction between my parents, which ultimately resulted in divorce. I was acutely aware of this discord. Their whole messy relationship affected me then and still does today.

By the time I first used drugs, I was a prime candidate for full-blown addiction. I loved them. They made my world bearable. When I started using cocaine, it was like finding God. It was like magic; I felt alive, beautiful, powerful.

A few years later, at age nineteen, I left home and became a model. It was then that my cocaine and drug use became high-maintenance abuse. The late 1970s were happening, and the motto was sex, drugs, and rock 'n' roll; a philosophy that I took to whole-heartedly. Life was a constant party. What was important was how you looked, who you were with, and what you had. I drowned my feelings of fear, insecurity, and self-hatred with huge quantities of cocaine, tranquilizers, and anything else that was available. I depended upon men for my self-esteem and for my drugs. They treated me like a small pet or a toy. That was fine, as long as they took care of me in the ways that I demanded.

As my cocaine use grew, it seemed that the party had ended for a lot of people. They continued on with their lives, but I couldn't stop. My world became strange and chaotic. I was holding on by my fingernails. It never occurred to me to stop using.

Picture this: I was living with a cocaine dealer. One night, three men broke into his apartment while we were there. They had guns and knives. We were tied up face down on the floor. One of them hit me when he caught me staring at him as he twisted rope around my wrists. They ransacked the apartment and put a gun to my boyfriend's head, threatening to kill him. Finally, after finding the coke and the money, they left, but not before I pleaded with them to leave us some cocaine. "Come on," I said. "There's enough for you to leave us a little." Although I didn't realize it then, something in me shifted a little; there was some small jolt of recognition of the fact that cocaine had become more important than my life.

I had moments of clarity throughout this time that terrified me. Suddenly, I would see what I was doing to myself, what was happening to me. Quickly, frantically, I would grope for my chemical escape. Physically I was deteriorating. My family didn't know what to do with me. Every time I talked to my mother, she told me I was going to die. My sisters had given me up for dead already. At the end, there was no one; even my dealer-boyfriend had dropped me, tired of the fights and of my stealing his stash.

I hated acknowledging my addiction. Initially it felt like a huge weakness, as if I had failed life in some profound way. I had. That was, and still is, hard to live with. It took some time before I listened and became teachable. There was much complaining and crying and fighting the Principles of the Twelve Steps. I went to meetings, took everyone's inventory, and did my distancing thing. Eventually, though, I started to get it. I heard the stories of others who, like me, had been to that dark, out of control, static place. They were laughing. They were changing their lives. I thought, "Damn, if they can do it, so can I." I have, too; slowly, haltingly, with my heart in my throat, dragging my feet like a reluctant child, but always with the sense that there is no other option. This is my life. I want to live it now, even if it hurts.

Cocaine Anonymous is now an important part of my life, but when I first got sober, C.A. hadn't yet been founded. I kept slipping in and out of other Twelve Step programs. C.A.

made an important difference in my recovery. At my first C.A. meeting, it felt like I had come home in some odd way. Sitting in a room full of people who knew what it was like to spend hours on their knees, either looking for bits of cocaine in the shag carpeting or staring fixedly through the keyhole, was incredibly comforting to me. There we all were, trying to grow up and take responsibility for ourselves, learning how to be participants in life, building the foundation some of us never had to begin with. I loved how hyper we were. Only recovering cocaine addicts are that crazy.

Recovering from my addiction and my past has not been easy. The process of self-discovery is a slow one. But, like they say: "Easy does it, but do it." And I do. On good days, life is an adventure, an opportunity to take back the power I gave away to cocaine and men, and I use it to make my life be the way it's supposed to be. I don't have a clue as to what that is, but I'm learning to trust in the process. I can make decisions now. I have choices. On bad days, I swear a lot and act like a brat, but I do not use drugs. I deal with the bad times; sometimes alone, sometimes with the help of others. I have wonderful friends and I've learned how to be a good friend in return.

My first reaction to the idea of a Higher Power was one of scorn and fear. I curled my upper lip and pictured Bible-thumpers doing their door-to-door thing. I am coming to believe a little more every day. Whatever it was I was searching for in all of those years of drug abuse had to do with the lack of anything spiritual or beautiful in me or in my life. I don't talk a lot about God — that subject is personal to me. I try to nurture that part of me privately, wanting it to become solid. Like everything else, it takes time — and time I have.

15

HE QUIT FAILING

He believed his life was doomed to failure, but in recovery he found that his old beliefs were all wrong.

*T*TOOK MY first drink of alcohol when I was thirteen years old. My father had died a year before, and I was uncontrollable. I had gotten by as a nonprogressive student by being the class clown. Now, nothing was funny. I stuttered. I didn't belong to any group. I was afraid of girls. But when I drank, I found something to be successful at: the other me. I couldn't read as well as anyone in my own age group, so all school work seemed to be harder for me than for anyone else. I was tutored through grammar school, but now I'd have it my way. I wasn't to take instructions from anyone for the next 30 years, except while incarcerated.

With school in the past, marijuana and I found each other. As a young man, I went to work in the film business. The use of alcohol and drugs was condoned, often preferred; life went well. The sixties found me with drugs, and money to buy more. I've heard it said that a person's worst day clean and sober was better than his best day drinking and using. That's not true for me. I loved drugs; they worked for a long time. I did it all: acid, ups and downs, mushrooms, peyote, booze, ether, morphine, and all combinations thereof. But cocaine — it cost more, worked better, and gave me what nothing else ever did. Eventually, it also took all that away, and more. You see, I did all drugs, but for the last eighteen years of my using, I drank as an alcoholic and used cocaine daily. I took drugs, traded drugs for friendship and relationships, and sold drugs for profit.

I moved around the country with my work and always found drugs available. My life was grand. With geographics a constant part of my life, and what seemed like everyone buying cocaine from me, it looked like a "no lose deal." Wrong!

Sometime during 1977, my drug use took a turn. I no longer desired to be sociable. I became paranoid. Worldly things no longer seemed to matter as much. I was constantly unhappy. Nothing felt right: not my house, my cars, or my nameless relationships. In 1978, I sold two pounds of cocaine to the D.E.A. My life turned into a shambles. They took everything and I was sent to prison. I adjusted well to the penitentiary. I drank and smoked grass daily. I was very popular with other inmates, staff, and correctional personnel. I was very progressive in prison. Even though I had graduated from high school, it was only by the skin of my teeth. I never learned anything, it seemed, except how to cheat and lie. Through testing in prison, I found I was dyslexic. I could not read or comprehend what I was being taught. I learned to read and write in prison. I yearned for cocaine every day.

When I was released from prison, I was bitter. My life had changed; I had lost so much. I tried to pick up where I had left off, to recoup. I floundered, it was over, but I wouldn't stop using. There were three dilemmas. The first of these was that I couldn't do enough drugs to bring that old high, that old feeling, back again. The second dilemma was that I was caught up in the penal system and, as with my addiction, I couldn't seem to get out. I'd violate my parole or get busted again and just couldn't stay out of jail. The last of these was that, with the first two things such a part of my life, I never got any worldly possessions back. Life just wasn't working.

I overdosed many times on a variety of drugs. In 1984, I spent nine days in a drug-induced coma. I contracted an affliction called Saturday Night Palsy: the loss of all use and feeling in the right half of my body. I needed physical therapy for a year. Still, I kept on using. I couldn't stop; though I tried. I started to care less for life. The last member of my family died. I was alone and felt it. Even though I was adopted at the age of two, no matter what problems I put my family through, no matter how my family abused me, there was still a bond. Now I was alone. This was the first, but not the most devastating, of many lonely feelings I would experience in the years to come.

Everything was futile now. Nothing was working. I was getting more irritable, irresponsible, violent, paranoid, and lonely. I believe no one knows loneliness like a cocaine addict on his way down. I carried a gun. I was never put in a position to use it, thank God.

In the middle of 1985, I either overdosed or, in a delirium, had tried to commit suicide. I spent seventeen days under observation in a hospital's mental ward. When I was released, I moved in with my dealer. For the next year, I watched, learned, and felt the demoralizing inconsideration that I had shown other people when I was a dealer. Now I had no foothold in self-respect, morals, or sanity. I spent all my time in a back room, alone and loaded.

I left this house, borrowed a little money to pay two weeks' rent, and moved into a weekly apartment under the pretext that this would help me go back to work. My spark was gone; I was unemployable.

Soon I was ducking the apartment manager; my rent had not been paid. I left the last of my possessions and took a bus downtown, a trip I made more and more frequently. This time I would not be taking the bus back. I found a way to secretly enter abandoned cement caverns; storage rooms located under Main Street. I walked a lonely, lowly path, head bent, lonelier than any man should ever be. I was beat up once by some street guys I didn't know. I remember waking one morning to find myself crying that I was alive. I met a transient who became a friend. He had been sober for six to seven months, and I had no idea why. He was an educated guy.

He told me that if I didn't get off the street soon, I would not be able to make that choice. I would become an accepted guy, then a man to know: "Prince of the Block," someone that was cool — what I always wanted to be. Then I would never leave. My friend convinced me to stop using and drinking and to get off the streets.

In the early fog of the last couple of years, someone who ran a recovery house had presented me with a chance to get sober. At that time, I was not interested. He had nothing I wanted. My response was rude, to say the least. Now, at the turning point, I knew what to do. I will be forever grateful.

With three days of sobriety, I called him. He still ran the same facility. He told me to be at the house the next day at 10:30 A.M. I left downtown that night. I walked for nine and one-half hours. As I walked, I dreamt of the new life I would have: just a simple little single room, and some day a car. I'd have a meaningless job, pay the electric bill, and be responsible. I knew I'd be lonely, but not as lonely. I'd be able to think; at that time it seemed as though I had no thoughts. Time would pass without my brain functioning at all. I thought of myself as "burnt" from drugs or "wet" from alcohol. I had been living for about two years in a bottom: not thinking, not caring.

Arriving Saturday morning at the rehab now seems like a monumental event. Then, it was a roof over my head, other people, food, and a place to be. I was greeted with what seemed like exuberance, as if they were expecting me. I shared a room with a using friend I knew from years before. Once on the property and settled into my room, I developed a fear of the outside world. Anything past the driveway was not safe. This fear had a smell, as did downtown and my living there. I was in a sanctuary. I feared leaving, even to go to meetings off the property. I would stay within touching distance of my roommates and the friends I had met at the house.

I remember, after I had been there a few weeks, some residents being told they had to leave, that room was needed for new residents. I can remember being tearfully afraid, begging not to be turned out, as I had nowhere to go. I promised to "produce" if allowed to stay. I was told to get my stuff and move into the garage. I was grateful. I produced; I stayed sober. I became willing to do whatever it took to embrace the program of Cocaine Anonymous. I stuck out my hand, walking through my fear of rejection. I was not sane. At times I would say things that would cause people to move away from me skeptically.

I became a worker of this Program immediately. I loved meetings, loved the Promises that were read, and believed the stories of the returning newcomers. I was certain my fate would surely be to end up downtown *alone* and *not die.*

I had never been successful, it seems, at anything until I found the C.A. program. It was as if it were invented for me. I immediately became friends with people whom I believed would stay sober; I ran with the winners. I read the Big Book. I had no trouble with my First Step. I ceased fighting the obsession to use, and it left me; after all, it had been a fair fight and I had lost. I was 43 years old. At this point, I found "hope," a new feeling in my life. I was home. I use the word "sanity" as my Higher Power. I had no God, and I knew my sanity was shaky. I prayed to "sanity" to pull me into itself. I acted myself into sane thinking. This act became habit and I felt myself being saved, returned to sanity.

I was allowed to stay at the same clean-living house for five months. I was grateful. I was told to get a job which involved no thinking. A job in a warehouse was created by an employer who years before had fired me for behavioral problems. I rode the bus to and from anywhere I went until after I took my first C.A. birthday cake.

I was on my way. Nothing mattered to me except going to

meetings and practicing the Principles the best I could. Like everything else I was told, this too worked. There was a thrill to being off the edge, to living life, to being humble.

I lived with other sober people until I was into my second year. I made Program friends. I went back to my old career and made clean friends there. Coworkers and friends from before were amazed. My life was on the move. Like I said: I was home, and my home was getting bigger.

Today, I'm a contributing member of Cocaine Anonymous, society, and the workplace. I've become the man I never wanted to be, and I love him. I love being responsible and caring for other people. I've had phone commitments at Central Office. I've been a panel leader and chairperson. I now sponsor several men. I have found a purpose in Cocaine Anonymous.

Let me tell you about just a few of the personal Promises that have come true in my life. I was a compulsive failure — I always knew I was going to fail which left me with constant fearful anxiety of the future. After getting clean and living a day at a time, I "came to believe" that I didn't have to have failure in my future. I stuttered all of my life from the age of four. I stopped stuttering after 40 years. I'm now back to work at a job I thought I was never capable of having. I now am the guy I used to work for. I quit failing.

I finished my Fifth Step with my sponsor at seventeen months sober. As I walked out of the room, he said, "How are you doing with relationships?" "Fine," I said. "I'm not having any." I was not only afraid of intimacy, I had become selfish with the results of living my life the way I had been. "Fine," he said. "Start to have some and start tomorrow. You're doing good." I had come to believe my sponsor knew what was best for me, especially if he's pointing out a character defect like selfishness and self-centeredness, or a fear like rejection. I started a relationship the next day.

That relationship turned into what is now my marriage of two and one-half years. My wife has several years clean and sober and is very active in C.A. She has a daughter who, like myself, is dyslexic. I love them both very much. My wife and I know that without sobriety, our marriage won't survive. We also know that we'll never keep what we're not giving away.

Thank you, Cocaine Anonymous.

16

STOP SIGNS

He rushed right past all the signs that said to stop using cocaine.

I WAS INTRODUCED to drugs while attending high school. It was the 1960s and drug use was rampant. Not wanting to be left out, I got high the first time drugs were offered to me. My gateway drug was marijuana and the high was so mild I wondered what all the hoopla was about. I experimented with a variety of drugs, never turning down anything that was around. I was vice president of the student body and associate editor of the school newspaper. I didn't view getting high as an escape; rather, it was an opportunity to expand my mind.

In my senior year I was introduced to cocaine. At the time, I didn't think much of it; the duration of the high did not justify the expense to me. However, I continued to use pot, pills, hash, beer, and wine into the early 1970s.

I went off to college and discovered amphetamines. At first the uppers were an "educational tool" or something to counteract other drugs or combat lack of sleep. While attending college, I married a nursing student, and my drug use took a new direction. In my junior year, I dropped out of college and got a job.

In the early 1970s, cocaine was the glamour drug. Not much was known about how dangerous it was. Coke was thought to be only psychologically addicting. I never thought of myself as addicted to anything, let alone to something as harmless as cocaine.

When my wife was a nurse, she had lost control of her life due to her addiction. She was stealing drugs from the hospital where she worked and injecting them. Wanting to keep her habit a secret, she used injection sites that were not obvious to the eye. She was finally caught, and panicked, and then fled the state to avoid prosecution. This incident confirmed my belief that I was not an addict, because I didn't use needles.

By the middle of the 1970s cocaine had become very popular. It seemed like coke was everywhere you went. Cocaine had crossed all walks of life and was readily available at work, at parties, and at bars. Even then, coke was not my personal drug of choice; however, I used it often. I started buying cocaine on a regular basis to share with friends at parties or in the parking lots of the bars where I hung out. I loved the illusion of prestige coke gave when I carried it around and everyone knew I had some. It's hard to remember exactly when, but at some point I gave up all other drugs and settled on cocaine. Those were the good years. I was chasing the feeling of those first coke highs, but could never quite catch them. I didn't know it then, but by the time I discovered that the illusion was a lie, the coke had turned on me. Cocaine would soon own me. I would do its bidding without remorse, and then deny that anything was wrong.

By the early 1980s, cocaine was an integral part of my life; it was no longer social or recreational. I never went anywhere or did anything without it. Every facet of my life revolved around the white powder that was constantly going up my nose. Cocaine was making all my decisions; it decided where I went, and who I was with. I began to ignore all areas of my life that did not involve cocaine.

A day came when I decided I would sell cocaine. I had illusions of money to be made, not to mention the status afforded to the man with the product. The reality was that I rarely made money, even after cheating friends and others with a short count. The truth was, I would use all the profits, promising myself I would make it up next time. Next time never came; I learned to freebase.

There's not much to say about freebase. I liked basing right from the start and could never get enough. When I reflect on those times now, I see it as an accelerated frenzy of self-destruction. There's no doubt that smoking cocaine hurried my descent to the bottom. Bad things began to happen to me that I didn't associate with the drug. During this period I married and divorced again. I had several live-in relationships which all failed. Not all of these women were addicts. The women who weren't addicts became frightened of what they were seeing, then left. The women who were addicts hit their own personal bottoms, then left. As for me, I just lumped them all into the category of "mistakes." I did not even have a clue that the problem was me and my cocaine addiction.

Looking back now, I see several signs that told me something was wrong. I call these "stop signs," events that would make a normal person stop what he was doing and examine what's wrong in his life. I was blind to these signs and others. More bad things began to happen to me; among them were four arrests, two for felonies. Some people might have stopped there, but I didn't. I remember an arresting deputy telling me that I was an addict whose habit had led him into criminal activity. I listened to what he said, but I didn't hear him.

As a result of the skill of a very good attorney, I was able to avoid going to prison. The attorney himself was a cocaine addict. We snorted lines off his briefcase in the court parking lot. The not-guilty verdicts enabled me to stay out there longer, denying I was an addict. I was, in fact, guilty of every charge, but I felt the police and the system were inept and that I could always stay one step ahead of them.

Those brushes with the law did have one ill effect. I had to borrow money against my house to cover my legal expenses. Money by that time was in short supply. The cocaine was devouring all my assets. I didn't bother to file income tax returns during those years. The I.R.S. caught up with me.

Between paying them and the legal expenses, I lost a house I had lived in for ten years. I blamed the loss on bad luck and made myself out to be a victim. I indulged in a lot of self-pity and was depressed most of the time. I had this feeling in my gut of impending doom and still I didn't stop.

My cocaine consumption continued to increase. I was using coke every day and was numb most of the time. I was in the middle of a week-long binge when my father died. I felt no sense of loss, no grief. I just went on using. Soon there would be another death with more disturbing implications.

I had befriended a coworker and we were very close. I was an only child and he was the brother I never had. I had introduced him to cocaine, and later he taught me how to freebase. Two months after the death of my father, my friend was found unconscious on his kitchen floor. He had been on a week-long freebasing binge. He was taken to a hospital and what followed was a nightmare from hell. At the hospital he was given a brain scan. I can still remember what the doctor told his family while pointing to the results of the scan. The doctor said: "The damage to this area of the brain is associated with heavy drug use. This damage is irreversible, he will never be any better than he is today." Twenty-six days later my friend died at the age of 36. During that time he went in and out of comas and lost sixty pounds of his body weight. I carried my best friend to his grave. I felt no pain, no remorse, no guilt or grief. I thought it was a bad break for him, that it could never happen to me. What was worse, I ignored yet another "stop sign."

I saved mention of my employment until last. The reason I did is because my job helped keep me in denial. Yet this was the biggest "stop sign" of all. I had the same job for seventeen years. I repeatedly told myself addicts didn't have jobs, let alone seventeen years at the same one. Addicts lived in alleys and slept in doorways or dumpsters, I told myself. My work record was excellent, not one mark against it. I worked as a trainman on a major railroad. I loved my job and going to work was fun. I fit right in and worked as a functioning addict for seventeen years, then something happened.

One day I arrived at my home terminal early in the morning. Instead of going home to rest, I partied all day. I went to a bar and began drinking and smoking with friends. Later in the afternoon, I went home and continued to party by myself. I went to bed at 10:00 P.M. At midnight, the phone rang. The scheduled time of my outbound train had been moved up. I had one hour to get to work. I was in bad shape and did several fat lines to pick myself up. I went on duty at the appointed time, not feeling great, but thinking I could make it. I reassured myself that, after all, I had done this kind of thing many times before. However, unknown to me at the time, things were going to be very different.

It was very early in the morning and very dark as our train left the city. We moved through the foothills before crossing the mountains into the desert. Suddenly, the interior of our locomotive was bathed in light; something was terribly wrong. On our track up ahead of us, was a railroader's worst nightmare, an oncoming train! At first there was disbelief, followed by panic and futile attempts to slow our train down. At this point, three things became painfully clear: collision was unavoidable, and no power on earth could stop what had been set in motion. Then came a sickening feeling in the pit of my stomach. I realized people would be killed or, at the very least, seriously injured. Finally, despite the fact I had lived my life as if it didn't matter whether I lived or died, I wanted to live. I did a very desperate thing to save my own life; I jumped off of a train going 40 m.p.h. into total darkness because I was afraid to die.

The two trains collided. The impact was earth-shaking, followed by the sound of bending, crumpling, and mangling of steel, as railcar after railcar left the track, littering the countryside with debris. The train we hit was carrying railcars loaded with automobiles that were now flying through the air and tumbling end- over-end. I thought to myself, "God make it stop." Because the crash site was so remote, it took the emergency equipment 30 minutes to arrive. I don't remember much of that time, because I was in shock. I recall climbing through that twisted and crumpled steel searching for the other crew members, terrified of what I would find. I remember looking at myself; seeing that my clothes were ripped and torn and covered with blood, but I couldn't feel any pain. I remember looks of astonishment on the faces of the paramedics that anybody could be alive. I was rushed to a hospital and treated for my injuries. Then I was given blood and urine screens, as mandated by law. I knew that I was in serious trouble.

Two months later, there was a hearing to determine the cause of the accident. The blood and urine screens had come back positive for cocaine, marijuana, and alcohol. At the end of the hearing, the blame was placed on the crew of the train I was on. My seventeen-year relationship with the railroad was severed on the spot. I faced a $250,000 fine and/or ten years in prison. So there I was, no family, no friends, no home, no money, no job, and facing a possible jail sentence.

I would like to tell you that that was the "stop sign" at which I stopped, but it wasn't. I continued to use cocaine for five more months. Only now, the using was different. I couldn't consume enough cocaine to make the emotional pain go away. I couldn't smoke enough to erase the nightmare of that oncoming headlight. They hadn't grown enough coca to fill the void inside of me. I was a shell of a human being. I knew I couldn't go on, and I knew I couldn't stop. I had to have help.

I entered a thirteen-month recovery facility, and it was there that I was introduced to Cocaine Anonymous. It was the people I met at C.A. who not only gave me the tools to go on with my life, but also the courage and strength.

I now have over 1000 days of sobriety. I have evolved into a completely different person. When I shave in the morning, I don't hate what I see in the mirror. I no longer have to lie, cheat, or steal to live. I have friends and our relationships are based on trust. Today I have a job. I am a contributing member of society, rather than a drain on its resources. My coworkers and friends see me as honest and dependable — someone they can count on. I no longer live in fear and dread of each day. Rather, I see each day as an opportunity to be better than the day before. Today I have a family that loves, cares for, and relies upon me. I have been awarded the custody of my two children.

The only fear I had of recovery was that I would be unable to have fun without using cocaine. Today I scuba dive, take white water raft trips, and enjoy other activities which allow me to actively participate in life. Today cocaine is not the center of my universe. I feel positive about myself. I feel that I have worthwhile contributions to make to my fellows.

There are rough spots from time to time, but C.A. meetings and the fellowship there smoothes them out. The C.A. meetings are where I go to get the material that fills that void inside of me. When I came into the Program, people told me not to leave before the miracle happened. As you can see, I didn't have to wait long. Every day I live in the miracle.

17

HAPPY, JOYOUS & FREE...FINALLY

A life-long search for acceptance led this young woman to a life of drug addiction, low self-esteem, and a feeling of emptiness. In C.A., she found not only true friendship, but also faith, hope, and happiness.

*W*HEN I WAS growing up, I believed what my parents told me, that I was family. Although I was unhappy as a child, I never questioned what they said. I thought my misery meant there was something wrong with me. None of us knew our family was dysfunctional.

We moved every one to two years throughout my life. I was always the new kid, the outcast, and I never fit in anywhere. I was attacked by strangers several times. My father had an unpredictable temper. Due to these and other factors, I learned how to shut down emotionally. I rarely trusted anyone. I developed compulsive behavior. I remember drinking as early as age three. I tried pot for the first time when I was twelve.

In the beginning of high school, I smoked pot to fit in with the cool crowd. Not surprisingly, I experienced instant popularity. I had finally found an identity. After that, my life revolved around getting high. Within a year, I was experiencing auditory hallucinations almost constantly.

I sincerely thought I was going insane, until I heard a commercial which described my symptoms and attributed them to prolonged use of marijuana. That scared me into quitting. After a year, however, I decided it would be okay if I smoked pot once in a while. I was wrong. Immediately after getting high I thought to myself, "Why did I ever quit? This is great!" I found myself right back where I had been the year before, and then some.

At seventeen, I tried cocaine. I don't remember enjoying the high, but I do remember thinking it was a cool thing to do. Shortly after that, we moved back East where the drinking age was eighteen. I found I could sneak into bars, and I really got into drinking. I also got into speed and sold it for extra cash.

After graduation I found an older crowd. I was the "baby"; they took care of me by giving me cocaine on the weekends. This went on for two years, until I decided to finish college out West. There I sold pot, using the money my family sent me. One of my clients was dealing coke. He wanted someone to binge with, so he supplied the coke, and we went on binges together for the next two years.

During this time, my parents took my younger sister to a rehab for an evaluation. The entire family was shocked when they admitted her. I flew there for my winter break. Family members who wished to participate were asked to sign a contract stating they would not drink or drug during this program. This created an enormous dilemma for me. After several minutes of contemplation and with tears in my eyes, I signed the contract. It was fortunate for me that I decided to participate. Although I remained in denial, I received a wonderful education. It planted a seed that would lead to my recovery four years later.

After I got home, I went on yet another binge, until it occurred to me that I would be graduating from college in a few months. I realized I might have to pass a drug test in order to get a job. I quit drugs for four months. After graduation, I got a job which had no drug testing. I was furious with myself for wasting four months of my life!

As was usual, that job lasted only two months. It was time for a geographic cure. I went back East for a visit. I discovered that most of my friends had become extremely involved with cocaine during the last three years. I went on a two-week binge that evolved into plans to move back East. I couldn't wait to get back to the party.

I sold nearly everything I had so that I could move. Afterward, I began a two-year binge. It was the beginning of the end. During this time, I did coke from Thursday to Sunday. I maintained control from Monday to Wednesday.

I met a coke dealer who repulsed me, but that didn't stop me from hanging around to get free coke. He gave me all the coke I wanted. In return, I was virtually his indentured servant. He would call me anytime and anywhere, and I would drop whatever I was doing to do his bidding. Often, I was running stupid errands or acting as liaison between him and his buyers. There were times I was put in dangerous situations in order to protect him or his business.

I did more and more things to get coke. I behaved in many ways I had always considered immoral. More importantly, I stopped enjoying coke, but I couldn't stop using it. This realization was my bottom. I continued this way for a year. I thought about quitting, but my exposure to coke was too great. Night after night, I promised myself I wouldn't do any, but the minute it came my way, I did it without thinking. Sometime near dawn, I would creep home. I would then spend the next several hours beating myself up over it.

During this year, I looked around at my friends. It was easy to see that their lives were unmanageable. It was very sad for me to realize that, since we had begun using coke seven or eight years earlier, my friends had turned into animals. All around me I saw my friends stealing from one another, trying to scam each other for drugs, lying, sleeping with each other's spouses, and gossiping about one another. My denial was too strong to recognize these things in myself.

I felt awful, looked terrible, hardly slept, and had daily nosebleeds, yet I couldn't stop. I knew I was physically addicted, but didn't think I was an addict. I thought there was a difference between physical addiction and psychological dependency. I said to myself, "Of course I'm addicted. Anyone who does this much cocaine is eventually going to get addicted." It didn't occur to me that someone who didn't have an addictive personality would never do so much in the first place.

I could see the sickness in my friends and knew I didn't want that kind of lifestyle. I decided to quit. I changed nothing in my life, except that I stopped using cocaine. Night after night, I watched my friends do drugs, and listened to them tell me that I was now a drag. It was torture. I caved-in to peer pressure after a month, and then binged for a month.

Thoroughly disgusted with myself, I quit again. This time I went to a Cocaine Anonymous meeting. I told myself I was going in order to give a friend support, when, actually, I was hoping to find help for myself. I could relate to a lot of what was said, but a lot of it scared me. Also, I didn't want to admit I was an addict, so I didn't go back. I managed to stay clean for three months on my own. Then came the holidays, and I binged through New Year's Day. After that, I decided to quit cocaine and alcohol. This time I lasted four months before I drank, and within a week I was back to cocaine.

After a couple of days on coke I became determined to quit. This time I stayed away from my friends. I spent the next four months in the deepest depression I have ever experienced. The emptiness I had always felt inside and my low self-esteem were magnified because I wasn't using anything to numb myself. Many days I never got out of bed. I wanted to stop living. Finally, I started trying several different Twelve Step programs.

I didn't relate to what happened there. I didn't meet many people because I isolated and didn't regularly attend meetings. I skipped from one meeting to another and from one program to another. I arrived late to meetings and left them early. I didn't share, and I hardly listened. I sat in the back. I avoided contact with other people. All the time I wondered why I wasn't getting it.

After a few months, I wanted to get it. I started paying more attention. But I felt like an outsider. Since I wanted to get the Program I was told "Fake it 'til you make it." So I tried that. I got a temporary sponsor and used her some of the time. I believed in meditating and I did that. Though I didn't believe in God, I prayed. I read most of the Big Book. I worked through the Twelve and Twelve, although I remained stuck on Step Two. Sometimes I read a daily meditation book.

I didn't pay attention to all the suggestions. I hardly used the phone at all. I didn't stop going to bars. I spent most of my time with people who were still using, rather than with people in the Program, and I didn't put sobriety first.

As a result, after nine months of sobriety, it hit me. I wanted to do cocaine again. I kept imagining what it would be like to go back out. This scared me a great deal. I knew I needed help or I would find myself back out there again.

Fortunately, a friend came to me and said she needed help getting off cocaine. I took her to the C.A. meeting I had gone to the year before. This time the meeting felt like it was my salvation. I felt at home. I walked into a room full of warm and friendly people — people who understood about cocaine. I recognized a few people from the year before, and this was very reassuring. That night I had plans to go to a bar after the meeting, but the people at the meeting invited me out for pizza. For once, I didn't isolate. They told me about other meetings and asked me to come back. I also got a few phone numbers. The cravings stopped and, before I knew it, the Program had finally gotten me.

I started going to six C.A. meetings a week, which I continue to do today. I finally started to see recovery work for me. For the first time in my life, I was happy with myself.

I discovered the nature of true friendship. In C.A., I made friends who cared about me for who I was, not for what I could offer them. My new friends were there for me when I needed them. They called to make sure I was okay. They gave to me but asked for nothing in return. It was hard for me to ask for help, but when I did, they were so willing to give it freely that asking became easier. No one in C.A. ever made me feel that I was an imposition to them.

I've lost the feeling of emptiness and loneliness that I carried with me my entire life. I had a hole inside of me that was as big as the Grand Canyon, and just as impossible to fill. This Program has banished those feelings. I haven't felt empty or lonely in sobriety.

The feeling of impending doom is gone. I always had a sense that something was terribly wrong. I constantly carried the feeling that disaster lurked just around the corner. Now I live with serenity. I know that everything is happening the way it is supposed to, that everything happens for a reason. This is the result of gaining the most amazing faith in a Higher Power.

Today, I am doing things I was never able to do when I was still using. I am living up to my own standards and morals. I am not ashamed of myself.

The two most important gifts I have received through this Program are faith and hope. Neither of them were a part of my life in the past. I had faith in nothing. I thought all that life had to offer was pain. Now I look forward to each new day. Every morning I thank my Higher Power for the opportunities that the coming day will bring.

Things still come my way that are difficult for me. But now I have coping skills and a support system to see me through them. I also have faith that everything will be okay, no matter what. It's not always easy, but today I see that life is a gift. I am enjoying the good things and overcoming the bad. I am enjoying people and allowing them to live as they choose. People care about me and I care about myself. At last I am happy, joyous, and free. My gratitude is endless. Everyday I try to remember what it was like out there and to say a prayer for the addict who still suffers.

18

FROM CANDY TO COCAINE

As a child, he used candy the same way he would one day use cocaine.

EVER SINCE I can remember, I was addicted to candy. I thought about candy constantly and had to have it with me wherever I went. I took it to school with me. I took it to bed with me. I took it to the dinner table with me. It was the most valuable possession I had as a child. I loved it, literally. I lived for it. I looked forward to the good feelings it gave me when I ate it, especially chocolate. It was chocolate I loved most. The best night of the year was always Halloween. It was like New Year's Eve to me.

During the summer, I worked odd jobs in the neighborhood, like mowing lawns and raking leaves. In the winter, I shoveled sidewalks and driveways to earn money. I sold my belongings to my friends, stole money from my mother's purse, and saved my allowance. I spent it all at the wonderful candy counter in an old corner grocery store at the end of our street.

I grew, and I got older, but I never grew up. Not much changed in my life, or in the way I related to life for many years. As a matter of fact, not much changed throughout high school or college.

Before I entered law school, I had never used drugs or alcohol in my life. I was always against those things, so I thought. Then, in law school I began to smoke pot and drink a bit. I enjoyed it. And so it was, through the time I graduated and entered the practice of law.

Then it happened: New Year's Eve, 1977. At the stroke of midnight, the girl I had a date with reached into her purse and pulled out a little vial. She looked at me and said "Happy New

Year, darling, this is cocaine, and we're going to celebrate."

For a moment, I protested. Then I hesitated. Then I tried it. From that moment on, my life was forever changed. I had traded in my childhood candy for adult candy. I had traded in Halloween for New Year's Eve. The addict had finally grown up.

At first, I was practicing law by day and doing cocaine by night. The two soon became one, and I didn't even realize it had happened. My life had begun to revolve around cocaine, just as it had revolved around candy as a child, and in many of the same ways. I had come to love it. I had come to live for it.

A friend and I bought a home in a nearby resort community. It was a place for me to get away, to ski and to mountain climb. The reality was that it was an excuse to get away to do more cocaine.

I couldn't stand people questioning me, telling me I didn't look good, and accusing me of taking drugs and of becoming irresponsible. Needing to protect my ability to use, I took more frequent and prolonged vacations, giving me freedom from family, friends, and business associates who just couldn't mind their own business.

One particular winter, I went to my resort home to spend a couple of weeks. When it was time to go home, I had a piece of cocaine I chose to leave behind for when I returned. For some reason I felt I needed to hide it, even though I was leaving it in my own home. I don't know why, but I always thought the whole world would be looking for my stash. So, I spent a couple of hours looking for the perfect place to hide my little piece of cocaine. I finally found the perfect spot. We were adding a room onto the house, and all that had been completed was the framework and the weather stripping. I decided on a particular place in the weather stripping and hid it there. I left and flew back home.

A couple of months later, I went back. When I arrived at the house, I found a surprise — the construction company had worked ahead of schedule, and had finished off the room. I mean *finished*. The plasterboard was up. The walls were painted. The paneling was up. The room was carpeted. Light fixtures were in place — the whole works. That room was a done deal. I remember saying to myself, "Well, there goes that cocaine."

That night I had a date with a girl and we stayed out very late. We did lots of cocaine. We finally ended up back at the house. In the middle of the night, we ran out of cocaine. I tried calling every drug dealer and friend I knew to get more, but without success.

I remember sitting on the couch with this girl, looking at her and saying, "I want to do more cocaine, and I know you want to do more cocaine, and there's cocaine in this house, but I can't get to it." I proceeded to tell her the story of how the cocaine ended up sealed behind the wall.

She just looked at me. With all the seriousness of a person making a critical life-decision, she said, "Well, couldn't we make just an itsy-bitsy hole in the wall?" What she said immediately began to make sense to me. I found myself walking out to the garage to get a crowbar. My mind was on automatic pilot. I was no longer a participant. I was an observer.

I had no idea where behind that wall I had hidden the cocaine; I was so high when I did it. But that didn't matter. I proceeded to demolish the entire wall, until I finally found that little piece of cocaine. It looked like a bomb had exploded, a huge pile of rubble with a crowbar lying on top.

It took us a little more than an hour to do the cocaine. And there was the wall, totally demolished. I had to hire the construction company to come back in and completely rebuild it. Yet I couldn't see it, my powerlessness — the insanity of my life.

Over the next couple of years, I saw more and more sunrises from the wrong side. I rarely slept. I rarely ate. I quit my law firm and became very isolated. I opened no mail, didn't answer the door, and didn't answer the telephone.

The inside of my home looked like an alley; empty bottles were everywhere. Tissue papers and paper towels were wadded up and thrown all over the place. Dirty clothes covered the floor. Food that I had ordered, but had never touched, sat rotting.

I would spend days just looking out the window, watching and waiting. I would also lie on the floor and watch under the door. I knew "they" were coming. I knew that "they" were out there. I would even pile-up furniture against the door to better protect myself from "them." I never knew who "they" were, but my paranoia was a living hell.

By now I had put so much cocaine up my nose that it ate a hole through my septum. I could have put a piece of string up one side of my nose and have had it come out the other side.

In the end, I spent nearly all of my time on the bathroom floor. I had been there for days. I had lost track of time and of the days. I had a large amount of cocaine to snort. I had always snorted my cocaine. I was bleeding profusely from the nose. There was blood on all the towels, blood all over the carpet. I couldn't stop doing cocaine.

Then something began to happen. I began to die. I had always experienced that feeling, like my heart was going to jump out of my chest, when I did cocaine. But this was different. I could feel the life going out of me. I began to lose control of all my faculties. I could feel myself dying. It is something you *know* when it is happening. I knew that I was going to die on that day.

I lay there on the floor, and in my view through the bathroom door, was the telephone, strung out into the hallway. I could see it, and in the worst way I wanted to crawl over to it, dial "911" and say, "Please, somebody help me, please send an ambulance!"

I did crawl. I crawled over to the cocaine and did more. At that moment in my life, using cocaine was more important than life itself.

I can only think of two reasons why I lived; one is because I ran out of cocaine, the other is that it was God's will.

That was in 1987, and it was the last time I ever used. I never allow myself to forget that day, or any of the other experiences which remind me of the powerlessness and insanity in my life. I need to remember where I came from. I need something by which to measure my growth.

I made it into this Program because someone else worked their Twelfth Step on me. Someone passed it on to me. Someone was out there after they got clean and sober, caring about others. I need to never, ever forget that. Had they simply gone on with their lives and forgotten about people like me who were still out there using and suffering, I wouldn't be here today. My gratitude begins with that fact. It is with that gratitude in mind that I reach out to others, especially the newcomers. I need to have them in my life. That is where my spirituality begins.

For me, spirituality comes from caring about others. I have found that the more I focus on improving the quality of the lives of others, the less I am into myself and my will. I feel a freedom and peace from within. The gifts I am beginning to receive in my life are greater than I could ever have imagined.

Something else I have done is that I have forgiven myself. I have forgiven myself for being an addict. I have forgiven myself for all the damage I did to my life, to my physical health, and to my career and finances. But most of all, I have forgiven myself for all of the horrible, negative, and unloving things I have felt about myself. It was not until I offered and accepted my own forgiveness, that I was truly able to grow in my sobriety.

Today I live a normal life. I don't take myself too seriously. Most importantly, my life is filled with lots of laughter, because I need to have fun. Sobriety has got to be fun for me. I am even able to laugh at my past. That is part of knowing that I have forgiven myself.

For me, this Program is about one thing — smashing my self-will and replacing it with spiritual will. I keep my faith in God and give him credit for the gifts and miracles in my life. And all I do is just keep showing up. I no longer think of life the way an addict does. I think of life as a human being does.

I am grateful to Cocaine Anonymous because I now have a choice in my life. I don't have to crawl over to the cocaine anymore. C.A. gave me the greatest gift of all: I got to write a happy ending to my story.

19

A LESBIAN GETS CLEAN AND SOBER

Today, she realizes that she can be a lesbian and not drink or use.

I AM AN ADDICT! It's such a relief that I don't have to use cocaine or any other drugs today, but it wasn't always like that.

My drinking started at the tender age of thirteen, when I was in intermediate school. On my way to gymnastics practice at 6:30 in the morning, I'd purchase liquor to drink on the way. I drank for the effect produced by alcohol. The effect, the high, the way I felt after any chemical was activated in my system, was what I wanted to feel.

High school was great. That's what it was to me, HIGH school. When I discovered I was a lesbian, my drug use increased. My new friends did drugs and I wanted to fit in. I smoked weed daily and had an occasional line of blow, too. I felt good and proud to be gay, and spoke out egotistically about being a lesbian.

My mother found out I was a lesbian when I was sixteen. We had a religious household, and it spared no room for a grave sinner like me. I left home and moved in with my lover. Living on my own gave me the right to drink whenever I was good and ready.

My lover and I moved across the country. I met a woman who was a hype; she stuck the first needle in my arm. From then on everything felt better coming from a rig. I quickly learned to hit myself, and my arms started tracking up rapidly.

Shortly thereafter, I discovered the pipe. The first hit scared me because I knew I was in for the time of my life. Before I knew it, my four hundred dollar weekly salary was spent on cocaine, but that didn't stop me; I'd do anything for cocaine.

I went on binges lasting three and four days. I wouldn't show up for work or even call in. I changed my circle of friends from users to dealers. I had to have cocaine in a big way. Many people got burned as a result of my expensive drug habit, and I had to move again.

I kept smoking, but my older brother was still slamming, so it wasn't long before I picked up that rig again. I'd go between smoking and slamming cocaine. I was very careful to clean out my set because I had gotten hepatitis before.

Money was definitely needed to support my habit, so off to work I went. One day I went in loaded and my boss and coworker Twelfth Stepped me. I started going to meetings to save my job. I went to a few meetings and took a couple of chips, but didn't believe those people were drug-free; they were always so happy.

I met a woman who fell in love with me. I was in so much denial, I didn't tell her I got high. I still thought I could stop or maybe hide it from her. However, it didn't take long before I disappeared to the dope house and stayed out all night. Upon my return, I had to get honest with this woman and tell her I was getting loaded. To my surprise, she wanted to try it. We were now both getting loaded.

It wasn't long before she started noticing that all her money was going up in smoke, and that we were not happy unless we were hitting that pipe. She threatened to leave me unless I got help and stopped using drugs. I tried stopping, but it was hard for me. I switched to using only weed and drinking every day. It still led me back to the pipe. Nothing could satisfy that passion for cocaine.

I thought of the meetings I'd attended and I found some Cocaine Anonymous meetings. Then my lover admitted me to a hospital for detox. I became a 30-day wonder, but got loaded ten days after getting out of detox.

I knew what I did was wrong so I tried again and stayed clean and sober for four and one-half months. Things didn't change: my attitude, my aggressiveness, the way I looked at things. My friends still used and I wanted to hang out with them. I dressed nicely, I looked good, and I memorized "How It Works," "A Vision for You," and the "Twelve Traditions." This, I knew, would keep me clean and sober.

The day came that I picked up again. You see, I thought I could hang around with my using friends and not use. I set myself up, thinking it wouldn't happen to me. My coworker smoked weed a lot and hit the pipe. I only hung around her when she smoked weed. The time came when I said, "Let me light that for you," and because I didn't get high, I thought it was okay. I lit another joint for her. Soon I had a drink, a beer with lunch. I thought, "Hey, I can do this and not hit the pipe." It was another week before I did hit the pipe. For the next few days, every waking moment, I obsessed on that next hit. The time had come when I was actively using again.

This spree lasted several months. I couldn't put together 30 days. I "came to" at a woman's house and had a moment of clarity. I wanted what those people were talking about and experiencing in the rooms of Cocaine Anonymous.

I begged and pleaded with the hospital program to let me back in; I was truly tired of living like I was living. My hospital stay lasted 32 days, and from there I was admitted into a social model Twelve Step program for 90 days.

This time it was different for me. I became teachable. I listened, instead of just hearing. I was quiet, quiet enough to hear a God of my understanding give me answers. I was of service, cleaning ashtrays I didn't even dirty. These were things I did because other addicts told me it was what they did to stay clean and sober. At a relapse prevention meeting, we discussed what the relapse trigger points were: fear, sex, anger, children, death in the family, having a lump sum of money. At that meeting we learned how to deal with those situations and that there are steps to relapse just like there are Steps to recovery. I had to focus on the Steps of recovery and beware of the steps to relapse.

My sponsor always encouraged the people she sponsored to stick together, to call one another, and to support each other. The time came, one day at a time, when I celebrated one year of continuous abstinence from all mind-altering substances. My new friends watched the transformation of a using, active addict into a happy, clean and sober addict in the process of recovery, as outlined in the Twelve Steps.

Today I assist addicts in the recovery process. First, I tell them to live their program like they drank and used. If they used every day, they should go to meetings every day. If they drove long distances to cop drugs, they should be willing to drive as far to get to a meeting. If they picked someone up to score some dope, then they should pick up newcomers and take them to meetings.

In recovery, I have learned something of utter importance to my personal and spiritual growth: my program of recovery must be an attraction for the newcomer, not a distraction. If I "thirteenth step" a newcomer, I am acting in an abusive manner. I must remember that the newcomer is vulnerable and willing to go to any length for recovery. They are not aware that getting sexually involved is a distraction from their own recovery. I feel we should teach them how to get and stay clean and sober; that is our purpose.

God is anything you want your Higher Power to be. However, remember not to get a Santa Claus-God. My ideas about a Higher Power change as I grow. My ideas aren't written in stone; they can, and will, change.

To the new person in the rooms or reading this book, or the person who keeps relapsing, I say to you, "Welcome. We've been waiting for you. You are very special. You deserve recovery. You deserve love. If you allow us to, we will show you what we did to get and stay clean and sober."

When I look at my life, I am truly grateful to God for giving me the gift of sobriety. My older sister died from drug use. My father died of a drug overdose and my big brother has tested positive for the HIV antibody because of his drug use. I've been spared from this, and it's my belief that I have a mission to carry the message that you don't have to do drugs anymore. There are ways to deal with life on life's terms without mind-altering chemicals. I have learned that Cocaine Anonymous has the solutions to my life's situations.

Thank you God and Cocaine Anonymous for saving my life. I am forever grateful for this gift.

20

THE HACK WHO BOTTOMED ON CRACK
Until God became his dispatcher, this cabbie could not find the road to recovery.

*C*OCAINE MAY NOT have been my first drug of choice, but crack was definitely my expressway to the rooms of Cocaine Anonymous.

I was like so many others whose drug use began while they were still teenagers. First I used alcohol, then pot, and then, a little further down the road, just about anything mind-altering. As I grew up in the late sixties, it was very much in vogue to tune in, turn on, and drop out. I wanted so much to be accepted, to be part of the in-crowd. I now see these attitudes as excuses to use drugs. My motto was "Live for today," not "One day at a time."

I quit school. I thought it was more important to have pocket-money for my extracurricular activities than to get a meaningful education. Of course, a conventional job was not for me. Nine-to-five jobs were just not cool. I found a job driving a taxicab, and it suited me just fine.

"What an ideal occupation," I thought. No alarm clocks to wake up to, no time clock to punch, and no boss. I got in a car in front of my home, and I was at work. If I did not want to work, no one missed me. If I needed money, I just put in more hours. I was the boss, and I was in charge.

All of this freedom made my job very enabling. I had no employer or employees to be accountable to. The boredom of waiting for fares and the anxiety of sitting in city traffic gave me plenty of excuses to use. If I had a great day, why not celebrate and get high? If I had a dismal night, why not feel sorry for myself and use some more?

Ultimately, I was turned on to such substances as heroin, cocaine, and crack, along with the places to obtain them. I had this notion that it was all right to smoke pot and to do blow while working, because they did not intoxicate me the same way alcohol did. However, pot slowed my senses, cocaine made me anxious, and both impaired my judgement. They may not have impaired it as much as alcohol did, but I sure got into my share of accidents. My addiction soon took me to even worse places than my occupation. Driving under the influence of any chemical was dangerous enough, but I also subjected myself to the dangers of picking up drugs in unlighted hallways and burned-out buildings. Sometimes I wonder why I am still alive today. Only God knows.

The realities of running a small business set in. Car, taxi medallion, insurance payments, taxes, and car repairs added up to a lot of financial obligations. The long hours these obligations demanded were stressful for me. I reasoned that smoking reefer was the way to deal with that. I needed cocaine primarily as a stimulant so I could put in longer hours and not be so fatigued.

Of course, the expense of drug use only added to my financial problems. After awhile, I used the excuse that the pressure from my lousy job was the reason I used. My job was what drove me to drink and use drugs. I couldn't figure out whether I used drugs to work or worked to use drugs. I failed to see that I was an addict. It was all an excuse to justify my usage. I was motivated by fear. I really feared having to find another occupation because I was afraid of dealing with life on life's terms.

I thought, like so many other addicts, that if I could change my circumstances, I could stop using, or at least curb my use. I was lonely and depressed. I felt the answer to my problems was to put an understanding woman in my life. My life seemed so empty because I had no one to love and to love me in return.

I met, and started a relationship with, a young woman who possessed a lot of the qualities I didn't have — qualities like being responsible and accountable. She had a good job with a lot of security, and that appealed to me. After a three-year courtship, we were married.

During that time, my coke use did decline and I became an occasional user. I really no longer enjoyed cocaine that much because of the anxiety and depression which resulted from its use. Coke also affected my sinuses, making them swell to the point that I could not breathe through my nose. This gave me sinus headaches. I continued to drink a little, but not while working. My pot use remained the same. Sometimes, to break the monotony of using marijuana, I would snort heroin to really get out of myself.

After three years of marriage, we had a child. I also thought this would curb my drug use. But now the pressure of raising a child, along with supporting my family and my bad habits, was even more overwhelming to me.

My life really started to become unmanageable. I worked all the time and was never home. This was how I hid my addiction from my wife. I was able to justify this behavior because as long as I paid all the bills, it was all right to do what I wanted. When my son was ten months old, my wife decided to return to work. It was not because she wanted to, but because she was not satisfied with the instability of my income. The deal was this: she would go to work during the day and when she came home, I would go to work. During that time in my life, I was not functioning very well. Being a mommy during the day and working all night, I got very little sleep. At the same time, crack was just becoming popular and was highly publicized in the media.

One evening, on my way to work, I cruised past one of my usual spots to pick up some reefer. My regular connection was hanging out, as always. He told me that not only did he have some dynamite herb, but he also had some crack for sale. I said that I was game and bought a dime. I mixed it up in a joint and liked the effect.

Several hours later, I went back for more. I told the street dealer how I had smoked it up in a joint and asked if there was another way to smoke it. He said, "Sure," jumped in the front seat of my car, and proceeded to show me how to use a stem. It seemed as though I was hooked immediately. I loved the rush and the instant high it brought. It didn't swell up my sinuses like snorting coke did. I was wired, wide awake, and ready to work through the night.

I have heard that "Insanity is doing the same thing over and over again and expecting different results." Crack became a vicious cycle of insanity real fast. As soon as the babysitter arrived or my wife got home from work to relieve me of my babysitting duties, I was out the door to go pick up. My cab seemed to be on automatic pilot when it came to getting to a crack house. I could not start work without first taking a blast. At first, nickels and dimes were sufficient to get me through the night. The problem was, I kept going back for more insanity.

The lies were also getting horrendous. I was always allegedly getting flat tires or having mechanical breakdowns. I would tell my wife how I had to wait three hours for a tow truck to come to my rescue, or how I was too tired to drive anymore and fell asleep in a rest area by the road. The lies were endless, just like my appetite for crack.

Even with all the pain I was in, I had no idea how to stop. I would disappear for days, and turn up at home all disturbed and distraught. I was always sweating, even in below-freezing weather. I suffered extreme weight loss and literally swam in perspiration in the oversized clothes I wore. My hands trembled so much that I could not even button my shirt. I either laughed hysterically or cried uncontrollably, for no apparent reason.

My bizarre behavior had finally become noticeable to my wife. I had hidden my disease so long and so well from her. I continued to con her. I told her that I was suffering from a great depression because I was out of work and had let her down.

One morning, after I returned from an all-night binge, my wife asked me if I would go with her to an outpatient psychiatric facility to see what was going on with me. Inwardly I knew the time had come. I was too sick and tired to argue. I was as beat as one beat addict could be. The elevator to my bottom was way past the basement. I didn't resist and went with her peacefully.

At the clinic, they diagnosed my depression as having been brought on by drug abuse. They referred me to a doctor whose expertise was in the field of recovery. He told me he had a good outpatient program. He said if I could be honest and willing to listen to his suggestions, I might not have to go away to a rehab. I feared having to go away because I thought my family would not be there for me when I returned. At that point, my wife was very upset and angry with me. I decided to start treatment immediately.

For the next couple of days, I had individual therapy and counseling. The following week I started group therapy. During the interim period I was to find a new job. I wanted employment as soon as possible because I had to get back on my feet financially, and I also knew that idle time might take me back out. With the classified section and God's direction, I found a job. At one time I didn't have enough confidence in myself to do anything but drive a cab. The job I found allowed me to put all my street knowledge to work in a positive way. My self-esteem was boosted so much that I felt elated and useful again. Continuity and routine were starting to take hold in my life, and I wasn't picking up.

In my outpatient therapy program, it was strongly suggested to get involved in a Twelve Step fellowship. I had not yet totally surrendered, and still insisted on doing things my way. I went to a couple of meetings and sat in the back. I didn't get a sponsor. I thought that therapy, my job, and my family were enough to keep me straight. I was wrong. I was told not to go to parties, but I did, and drank. I was very much in denial about my alcoholism. Whenever I drank, I got drunk, even when I drank only beer at a ball game.

After the initial fog had lifted, and the pink cloud had burst, I still thought pot and booze were accepted vices. I failed to see the progression towards my total devastation, which was crack.

I soon learned that the disease of addiction is three-fold. In my case, the three folds turned out to be Thanksgiving, Christmas, and New Year's.

My wife was very instrumental in my recovery. I believe that God works through other people, and I am sure my wife was chosen by God to show me the way to a drug-free life. There was some confusion on the matter that alcohol was also a mind-altering drug. We did our usual entertaining over the holidays with family and friends. Unfortunately, there was always alcohol in our home and at the other functions we attended. With the rest of the family drinking, I found it acceptable to drink also, especially since I was not condemned for it like I had been for my drug use.

After Christmas, an old friend showed up at my home. He was one of my old pot-smoking buddies, and I knew for sure he had a few joints with him. I had been drinking, so I thought, "What harm would there be if I smoked a little reefer?" We went out for a ride in his car where we smoked some marijuana. When I arrived home, high and glassy-eyed, all hell broke loose with my spouse. "How could you go and use?" she cried out, not realizing I had been using all along in light of my recent drinking. "I am leaving you. We're through!" she screamed. "Better yet, I'm throwing you out. Tomorrow I am going to see a lawyer about a divorce."

I became very emotional. Feelings of embarrassment, guilt, and shame resurfaced. I couldn't blame my wife for being angry, nor could I blame her for making me use. I can only thank her for helping me realize how wrong I was for using, and awakening me to the fact that using any mind-altering substance would sabotage long-term sobriety.

Fortunately, I talked my wife into seeing a marriage counselor instead of an attorney. The counselor explained to us that the disease of addiction affected us both, and that a concerted effort must take place if we wanted our marriage and our lives to improve.

I have not had a drink or used a drug since, even though I spent that New Year's holiday very unhappy, with feelings of self-pity and anger. Thank God a miracle was soon to happen!

A new year had just begun, and there was plenty of hostility in our household. On top of that, my mother became very ill and had to be hospitalized. One Sunday, my wife and I had an argument. I stormed out of the house in a rage. I went for a ride in the car, hoping this would calm me down. When I gained some composure, I decided that I would go visit my mother in the hospital. Upon my arrival, I found the main entrance to the hospital closed, and was directed to use an alternate entrance. After entering, I noticed some people seated in a classroom. I looked into the room to see what was going on. To my amazement, I saw the Twelve Steps and Twelve Traditions hanging on the wall. It was like God showed me the way to this room. To me, this was the spiritual experience I had to have. It turned out to be a Cocaine Anonymous meeting.

I identified with the feelings and the stories of the people at the C.A. meetings I started to attend. I found comfort there and finally felt at ease and at home. I started to follow suggestions as directions, and most importantly, I kept coming back.

It then became apparent to me that I had a decision to make. Was I to keep on using and die in the hell of addiction, or would I take certain steps and live in the heaven of recovery? Thank God I chose the latter.

Today I realize that there are no coincidences, they are just God's way of remaining anonymous. Now I don't get high because of that channel they talk about in the Eleventh Step prayer: using drugs only puts static on the frequency and makes it harder to have a conscious contact with my Higher Power. Life has become a spiritual journey, and only with God's power can I stay clean and sober.

At one time, I got a lot of satisfaction when people told me what great drugs I had. That satisfaction does not compare in any way to the overwhelming gratification I feel today when I am complimented on my growth in sobriety. Today I know a new freedom because the Promises they talk about in the Program have become a reality. I now have ambition, virtues, and values in my life. I have a Higher Power. For all of this, I am forever grateful.

21

THE MIRACLE OF RECOVERY
She found recovery in spite of herself.

I WAS FIRSTBORN of five children. Mom had all of us in a six-year period. In her seventh year of diapers, formula, and sleepless nights, she kind of changed. I then had to assume a lot of responsibility. It was years later before I understood the concept that our disease was a family disease. My mother suffered considerably.

My dad handled all of this by becoming one of the most functional alcoholics to ever exist. He was good at it; he had to be. His job was running the family-owned business. His father was his boss. Grandfather was also a two-fisted drinker when he wasn't using those fists to teach his sons lessons in responsibility. Dad was at work every day. He was responsible and functional and worked to keep his five kids fed and clothed. He doesn't sound like an alcoholic does he? However, his binges were legendary, as was his sense of shame. He hated himself after the binges and the trouble: the fights with my mother; the police escorts home; his family seeing him in the pits of a hell he could not control after picking up the first drink.

My father quit drinking nine years before he died. A doctor made a wager with him, and put his money on Dad's liver quitting before Dad could quit drinking. He quit, and won the five bucks, but you never met a more miserable man in your life.

Off and on for quite a few years, eighteen years to be exact, I would go to a Twelve Step fellowship in which the only requirement for membership was the desire not to drink alcohol. It said nothing about the cocaine or other drugs I was using. My own ability to justify, my dishonesty, and my denial that cocaine was a problem kept me from utilizing that wonderful program. It was Cocaine Anonymous and its Third Tradition: "...a desire to stop using cocaine and all other mind-altering substances" that took away my loophole. C.A. called my bluff.

Cocaine seemed the answer to all my problems. I wasn't tired anymore. There were no nasty hangovers, no throwing up at inopportune times. I could also play chemist and mix it with other drugs for whatever effect I had in mind. What more could I ask for? I even became a business tycoon of sorts, to get my coke at no cost. At least it seemed like no cost, until I found myself doing time at a women's correctional facility. By this time, besides going to jail, I had lost my children, been in hospitals for overdoses, been in mental institutions, detoxed at various clinics, gone through three marriages, and tried to commit suicide; not to mention all the psychiatrists, psychologists, therapists, and counselors I managed to visit.

I just could not make the connection. How could the substance that made me feel like I knew I was supposed to feel be a problem? I was positive I was born with a chemical imbalance, and I knew adding cocaine balanced me right out.

With cocaine I had charm, poise, confidence, and beauty. People could finally recognize my true talents. With an eight ball I was "Queen for a Day." Oh sure, sometimes your supply gets dangerously low and you can't find your connection. You get nervous, tense, and a bit irritable. You may feel less than perfect at times because of a bit too much or a bad cut. I would achieve what I like to call "the perfect plane of paranoia": flying to windows to see who's looking in; to closets because you know someone's in there, just waiting for you to leave; and to check out those trees and bushes, which *are* moving closer to the house. My favorite is the "someone-is-in-the-back-seat-of-my-car-while-I'm-driving-I-must-stop-wherever-I-am-and-run" feeling. But you have to understand that without the drug, it was worse. If cocaine wasn't available, anything that could change my reality would do. Sober reality was my nightmare.

Before I started using drugs, if I walked into a room, no one in that room looked as insecure as I felt. I was plagued by guilt, shame, anxiety, remorse, and hopelessness. I suffered from my own unique type of loneliness. It seemed that when other people were lonely, they called a friend and felt better. When I was lonely, I was already convinced I had no friends. I would sink into a depression and isolate completely. Self-pity would set in. Eventually I just knew I was losing my mind. I experienced a sort of free-floating anxiety. I spent a lot of time waiting for "it" to happen. I had no idea what "it" was, I just knew "it" was bad. I would come to the point that I wanted "it" to happen just to get "it" over with. I felt persecuted, haunted by the past, fearful of the present, and terrified that the future would be no different. I made more attempts at suicide before I started using drugs than at any time in my active addiction.

I made the rounds of the medical community, trying to find the magical cure for my problem. I would explain the problem and get the appropriate pill to relieve the symptoms I listed. I would use it, magically feel better in a few days, and know I was cured. To celebrate, I would buy some cocaine. I always knew there was something wrong with me. I felt that if only whatever it was could be cured, I could then use drugs and not get so carried away. Usually I was literally carried away to another hospital.

Of course, I had to eventually come to the realization that this was insanity. I was called crazy enough times, by enough people, that I felt I owed it to myself to check it out. My insecurity was enough to convince me "they" were right.

Now, don't get me wrong. I have great admiration for the psychiatric community. If I had been mentally ill, perhaps they could have helped me, but I am an addict. All that the psychiatrists, psychologists, therapists, and community counselors did was give me reasons to justify my behavior. It would go like this: at some point in my therapy, as I was listing my numerous complaints, my continuous bad breaks, and the details of my rotten lot in life, the therapist would interject with something like, "You mean to tell me you raise these children by yourself, with no support from your family?" I'd be real brave about it in front of him and go on about how much I sacrificed for my babies.

I'd start thinking about it on the way home. Other mothers have a husband to help relieve some of the pressure of being with the children all day. Did I? Noooo, not me. Other moms had their mother to help, who *wanted* to spend time with their grandchildren. Did my mother? Noooo, not her. All she did was crab about what a rotten mother I was. I was convinced I was a victim, felt very sorry for myself, and knew I deserved a break. So I would stop for "just one." The compulsion would set in, and I'd be off again. Three days later, I would be wondering where those children were for whom I had sacrificed so much.

It was not until I was hospitalized the last time that anyone pointed out that it was my selfishness, my self-centeredness, and my desire to reject responsibility that was the big problem; I was the problem.

The miracle of recovery came as quite a shock to me. I was on my way to see my connection. I had two bottles of frozen vodka with me. I made my score and stopped to have a taste before going back to town. The next thing I knew, I was "coming to" in a clinic, wondering where I was. I was so sick. I couldn't remember ever being so sick and afraid. I had lost my children, my home, my car, and all my belongings. I had no money, no friends, and no family — again!

As soon as I was well enough, I threw a stupendous "pity-party." I moped, I cried, I did everything to try to get out of the situation. This was my normal routine whenever I found myself bottomed-out. Usually some good Samaritan would pat me on the back and tell me, "It will be fine dear, don't you worry." Shortly thereafter, I would be using them for all they were worth. This time though, it was different. First of all, I never got mentally defogged enough to run my usual con. Today, I choose to believe that it was God, doing for me what I could not do for myself. He did not let me run my con. He kept me in that fog until, in spite of myself, I started to recover.

One of the first things I realized was that I had no idea how *not* to use drugs. I wasn't so sick that I could not remember how miserable I could be when I was straight. I moaned about that until a recovering cocaine addict said to me, "Stop your moaning and being so damn selfish. Obviously you need to work this Program or you wouldn't be here." No psychiatrist had ever talked to me like that. I probably would have fired him if he had; he would have been too close to the truth. This addict told me the truth for free. He may have saved my life. How dare he talk to me like that! I was going to work his damned Steps out of spite now!

I used to compare stories I heard in meetings and think, "I wasn't that bad. I guess I'm not one of them." I spent a lot of time wishing I had quit after the first hospital stay, or the first trouble I got into. It took working the Twelve Steps to realize that I could only recover from my disease if I worked the Program. I had to be at the crossroads and willing to go to any length to recover. When you can't be high, and are miserable sober, there is only one way to go: get willing to trudge that road to happy destiny. I can guarantee you one thing: if you have lost it all, or if you have only gotten a slap on the hand, the Twelve Steps of Cocaine Anonymous can only improve your life. You can never lose.

I admitted that I was powerless and that my life was unmanageable. It didn't take a rocket scientist to see that. I was able to admit my insanity after hearing someone say, "Insanity is doing the same thing over and over, and expecting different results." The only thing I had never tried in my life was the Program. I figured by then that anyone could do a better job than I had. What did I have to lose? Next, at Step Three, I created my own God and gave Him my will and my life.

What I lost by working the Steps was my arrogance, selfishness, fear, confusion, paranoia, anxiety, despair, denial, and dishonesty. I have peace of mind, and that is the greatest gift. All I had to do was tell God and another human being about me. I asked Him to make me honest and, therefore, more tolerant. I told people I was sorry for things I had done, even if I felt they'd screwed me. I checked my progress every day. I prayed and meditated, on my knees, because being humble is hard for me. Then I carried the message of the gifts I had received to other addicts who still suffered.

It was not as hard as I'd thought. Though it had taken me a long time to get sick it has only taken two years and nine months to feel this good. What a deal!

I just got a great job doing what I do best, helping my recovery by asking God to help me help someone else. I have all four of my children today, and I always know where I left them. Sometimes they even know where I am. I have a daughter who is graduating high school this year. Another daughter works her own program of recovery, as the child of an addict. My son is simply my son, and today I don't have to get cranked over him getting dirty when he plays. Then there's my baby, whose younger years I have been able to experience sober.

One more thing: the loneliness. It's gone. The First Step says, "We admitted," and as soon as you admit that you are powerless, you become part of that "We." I may not have family here, but I have friends who are all the family I need. I have a best friend. That may sound dumb, but I never had one before. For the last two years, we have had a running feud and have taken every available opportunity to point out each other's character defects and shortcomings. But when I had to be hospitalized over the summer for surgery, that man moved into my house and made sure my children ate and were cared for. Try getting that kind of love from your coke connection!

I am grateful I'm an addict. I have been given a chance to be reborn, to live, to love, and to laugh. God gave me C.A., and Cocaine Anonymous has given me a life I am now grateful to live.

22

A STRANGER IN THE MIRROR

God was working on a miracle for this young woman before she realized she needed one.

*T*AM NOT one of those people you hear say in meetings, "When I walked in the doors of Cocaine Anonymous I knew I was home at last!" My first Twelve Step meeting was like a bad date after which you hear yourself tell him or her:

> "Gee-I-had-a-REAL-interesting-evening-Thanks-for-sharing-the-gory-details-of-your-life-with-me-but-no-I-don't-think-we-should-do-it-again-sometime-soon-because-we-really-have-nothing-in-common."

Get the picture? Denial at its deepest. You see, at my first meeting, while in a rehab, I was seated between a nine-months-pregnant woman with base pipe burns around her mouth and her boyfriend, who was blinded when that same pipe exploded in his face. The speaker of the meeting was a fifteen-year-old ex-hooker. She shared about how she had been gang-raped while turning a trick at age twelve so she could make money to support her crack habit.

Three years earlier, I had stopped using cocaine and substituted intramuscular narcotics, tranquilizers, and prescription pain pills. Alcohol had never interested me. I still had my eyesight, the house on the beach, and the red convertible. I wouldn't have called myself a coke-whore if my life depended on it. (Although a few years earlier, I *had* developed an attraction to the cocaine the undercover narcotics officer I was sleeping with was skimming from his busts.) What I didn't have was the $250,000 I owed various hospitals because of my pain shot abuse, my husband who had left me for another woman, and my sanity, long-since gone. I couldn't relate to anything I heard shared, because I was listening for the differences rather than the similarities in the stories of the people I heard sharing. I was *real* happy those poor souls had a place like C.A. to go to. I couldn't wait to get the hell out of that room and pop a few of the tranquilizers I had smuggled into the hospital.

I had a few good reasons for checking into a rehab: I was walking into walls and hallucinating. Most importantly, I was hiding from my husband whom I had falsely accused of spousal rape the day before. All I wanted was to detox for a few days, get my head clear, and work on getting my husband back from "her."

I managed to stay drug-free for 57 days before relapsing on tranquilizers and self-pity. The tranquilizers led me back to pain shots and week-long binges. I would go to dozens of hospital emergency rooms within a 200-mile radius of my home and con doctors into shooting me up with any type of narcotic I could get for my imaginary back pain. I had already had two back surgeries and knew how to "hurt" convincingly. When my back pain stories wore thin on the doctors, who were beginning to see through my ruses, I began to "suffer" abdominal pains. I had three surgeries I knew I didn't need; two of gynecologic nature and... well, I heard you really didn't need your appendix anyway. I figured that surgeries guaranteed pain medication every three hours, 'round the clock.

The day came when the drugs stopped working. The emotional pain could no longer be numbed by downers. Thoughts like: "I'm not good enough," "I'm not worthy of love," and "I'm useless," tormented me.

I heard that my husband had violated parole and was back in jail. I had married him one year before while he was incarcerated. We had the perfect marriage for an entire year because I knew where he was at night; I was that insecure. I just knew that, although the Twelve Step program did not work for me, it would work for him! I figured the best way to get out of my depression was to carry the message to my husband and, at the same time, try to win him back. He was a captive audience, and I liked it that way.

I took my Big Book with me and paid him a little visit. Imagine my surprise when he wouldn't talk to me! I guess he was still a bit miffed about that spousal-rape charge. I watched as he and his girlfriend shared some intimate chatting. I went dead inside. It hurt to see them together, but I had to watch. Then I began to seethe. I followed her into the jail parking lot, got into my huge sedan, and watched as she got into her tiny subcompact. I followed her onto the freeway and promptly ran her car into the center divider at 80 m.p.h.

Luckily, she wasn't hurt and didn't prosecute me for attempted murder. I sunk deeper into debt, depression, and drugs. The bad feelings, resentment, and despair wouldn't go away. I knew that I would seriously injure somebody if I didn't lock myself up somewhere. I had hit bottom financially, mentally, emotionally, and spiritually. I begged a God I didn't believe in for a miracle.

Desperate for anywhere else to go but home, I checked back into rehab. I recall looking into the bathroom mirror of my hospital room and being shocked at what I saw. There was a stranger in the mirror. A severely underweight 60-year-old woman, with gray skin and sunken eyes, was glaring back at me. What made it so shocking was that I was only 25 years old. My reflection had no soul. I figured that I had nothing to live for and no hope for recovery. I felt that since my soul had died, my body might as well follow, so I slashed my wrists.

I found myself in the locked mental ward of the hospital an hour later. I had accidentally set off the emergency buzzer on my way down to the floor when I collapsed.

Everything sharp was taken from me. The hospital staff left me only a Big Book to read. I guess they figured I wouldn't be able to find a way to kill myself with it. For lack of anything else to do, I read the first 163 pages. On page 164, where "A Vision for You," as heard in meetings, can be found, the room lit up with a flash of sunshine. For the first time in my life, I felt the presence of God. There, in the last two paragraphs, was my miracle.

The Twelve Step program is explained in "A Vision for You" in the simplest of terms. I had heard it a hundred times in meetings, yet had never listened to it. I understood at that moment that I had to work the Steps and change, or I would die. My psychiatrist walked in just then and told me that since I was a danger to myself and others, I was being transferred to the state mental hospital in fourteen days. I told him of my spiritual experience and pleaded with him to let me transfer back into the chemical dependency unit of the hospital. It did no good. I accepted the fact that I was going to the state mental hospital, no matter how spiritual I was.

I noticed that the sunshine that had flooded the room earlier was replaced by darkness as storm clouds gathered overhead. I cursed God for making it rain. I was depressed enough as it was. It rained for two days, nonstop. I was awakened on the third day by a nurse who ordered me to pack my things. I was a bit confused because I wasn't supposed to be transferred for several days. I asked her what was going on. Her reply was like music to my ears. She said, "This wing of the hospital is under six inches of water from the rain. We have to move you into the chemical dependency unit where it's dry, or the Health Department will shut us down." I swore I would never again curse God for bad weather.

I was to be on a form of probation for the remainder of my stay, or the state mental hospital would become my new home. I enthusiastically attended the first C.A. meeting of my new recovery with bandaged wrists. I took a newcomer chip, sat down, and for the rest of the meeting listened for the similarities and ignored the differences. I made Cocaine Anonymous the Fellowship of my recovery, even though I had stopped using cocaine years before. I love the way the C.A. First Step reads: "We admitted we were powerless over cocaine and all other mind-altering substances — that our lives had become unmanageable."

I immediately told my physicians that I was an addict and could manipulate drugs from them. I explained that my body didn't know the difference between drugs for pain and drugs for pleasure, and that I could fake pain without realizing it.

I then set four goals for myself to reach in the first year of my sobriety. I accomplished every single one. I filed for bankruptcy, found a job, and made amends to my husband's girlfriend. My fourth goal scared me but proved to not be as painful as I thought. I made amends to my husband, and allowed him to go ahead with divorce proceedings. I learned that rejection is God's way of telling me that someone doesn't belong in my life.

I attended lots of meetings and kept a journal of all the experience, strength, and hope I heard shared, read, and discovered on my own. I referred to this journal of quotations whenever I thought I couldn't make it another day. When suicide seemed more palatable than getting loaded, this journal gave me inspiration to go on. I found that when all I can handle is a 10.0, God throws me a 9.99 — I am never given more than I can handle. Tough times happen in sobriety, but they soon pass.

I have found that in working the Twelve Steps of Cocaine Anonymous, I had begun living the Principles of the Program without realizing it. Step One taught me honesty and acceptance. I had to get honest with myself and admit I had a living problem, not just a drug problem. Only after admitting this was I able to accept my circumstances and look for help.

I learned open-mindedness and hope by working Step Two. The hope came from seeing other recovering addicts getting better who had come from a place similar to where I had been. Being open-minded allowed me to discover that the world did not revolve around me! When I realized this, I was able to find a Power greater than myself.

The Third Step taught me faith. It proved to me that "God could and would if He were sought." In Step Four I made a searching and fearless moral inventory of myself. Not him. Not her. Not them. But me! This Step required courage that I had to pray to receive. The courage I was granted enabled me to look at my past. From there I discovered that action would be needed if I was to prevent myself from repeating the same mistakes. I found that inventories are great pain relievers and learned that pain repeatedly experienced indicates a need for self-assessment.

I shared my inventory with my sponsor and God in Step Five. I learned integrity in the process; integrity gave me the dignity to be able to hold my head up high. When I shed light on my fears and admitted my transgressions, they disappeared like shadows, and I was set free. This was the point at which my self-esteem began to return.

In Step Six, I listed my character defects, including my obsessions with people, places, and things because they are one and the same. It took a few hours because I had so many "survival skills" to write down. I was afraid that removal of my defects would also remove my personality. But I knew that the principle of willingness to change which accompanies this Step was for my own good.

I learned a lot about humility in working Step Seven. I had thought that I would wake up perfect the day after I prayed to have God remove my character defects. Not so. I found that my Higher Power has a sense of humor. He lets me see myself indulging in inappropriate behavior until I can't stand being me and beg Him to take away whatever defect I am practicing at the time.

I took the list of people I had harmed from my inventory. I saw where I was wrong and prayed for willingness to make my amends. The people I thought had wronged me didn't seem so bad after I had prayed. I was shown brotherly love in the Eighth Step, which is respect for my fellow man.

Step Nine required sound judgment in the process of settling my debts. A debt is a situation requiring forgiveness or reparation for insult, injury, or loss. In making my amends, I sought to settle my debts without stirring up pain or trouble for others. I swept my side of the street clean and found forgiveness. I was also able to rebuild a few bridges I burned.

Step Ten taught me perseverance and discipline. I must work my program on a daily basis in order to grow steadily. I keep tabs on myself by reviewing my day with a nightly personal inventory. I list not only the defects I experienced during the day, but also my assets. I make amends as soon as I am aware I owe them. A nightly inventory helps me keep balance in my life.

The Eleventh Step has taught me spiritual awareness. As I constantly seek to improve and expand my spirituality, I find I am becoming more intuitive. I start each day with a prayer that I may do God's will for me and I meditate for knowledge of that will.

Step Twelve is about service and learning how to contribute to the lives of others. It's about unlearning selfish ways. I abused friendships and took from others all my life while thinking that the world owed me something. Service work is how I give back what was so freely given to me and how I express my gratitude to Cocaine Anonymous. By practicing the Principles and sharing about them with my fellow addicts,

I get back ten times what I give.

I would like to end my story with the four paradoxes of recovery as I have come to understand them: I can't keep what I have unless I give it away. I had to surrender to win. I had to suffer to get well. I had to die so that I could live. This last paradox reminds me of the stranger in the mirror. She had to die after all, and I couldn't be happier!

23

A COUPLE OF SURVIVORS

Their relationship was filled with love, respect, and friendship — until cocaine ripped through their lives. Only the power of C.A. could restore their relationship and allow them to survive.

HE MIRACLE OF our story is that we are alive and still together to be able to write it. You see we almost didn't make it — neither as individuals nor as a couple. Since our relationship and our lives, which were destroyed by cocaine, were put back together by Cocaine Anonymous, we felt compelled to share our experience as a couple. Our message is that there is hope — no matter how bad or hopeless life seems, it can get better.

It wasn't always bad with us. In fact, we had the best and greatest relationship any two people could ever have. We met in a bar, as all good addicts and alcoholics should. From that day, until thirteen years later when we walked into this incredible Fellowship, we never spent a sober day together. It was a match made in heaven. If I smoked a joint, my wife would say, "What about me?" Then she would join in. If I was doing some coke, that cute little voice would pop up and say, "What about me?" That's the way it went. It was me and "What about me?" — joint-for-joint, pill-for-pill, toot-for-toot, and, in the last three years of our using, base hit-for-base hit. Sharing all the other drugs was never a problem. But when both of us were freebasing coke, sharing was no longer fun. It was more like — "Give me that pipe, you selfish S.O.B.," "It's not your turn, it's mine," or "Is that all you're giving me? I want more!"

Smoking coke became the most important thing in our lives. When we were bingeing we missed work, neglected our daughter, and wouldn't even answer our phone. Basing was all we thought about. We would go to the movies and watch the titles at the beginning, then look at each other and say, "Let's go get the pipe," then leave. We would be getting dressed to go out to a party or some other function, one of us would pass by the other, and our eyes would meet. Smiles would come across our faces and we would say, "Why don't we do just one hit before we go?" Famous last words: "Just one hit." That "one hit" could go on for three hours or three days. We never really knew. We became famous for being late. People would always tell us to arrive at 7:00 P.M., even though everything would start at 9:00 P.M.

I remember one Mother's Day when I was trying to decide what I would get for my wife and I finally thought of the perfect gift. I got her a custom made base pipe and a blowtorch. She loved it!

We had no idea that we were headed down a road from which there is no return, especially for a marriage or a relationship. No matter how much two people love each other, cocaine and the pipe always become more important. And we did love each other. Before we started our "social" basing we were the happiest and most loving couple that you ever met. We had respect and trust for each other and open communication. We had a baby, a little girl, and life was great. We just did some grass and ludes on the weekends. Looking back at it all, we appeared to be a "normal" family. In fact, neither of us came from homes where drugs or alcohol were a problem. Our parents didn't drink or use drugs. Our home lives were basically loving ones. People would have never thought we would end up doing the "low crawl" on our shag carpeting looking for any coke or rocks we might have dropped, like desperate lunatics.

As our disease progressed and the using increased, all of the love, respect, trust, communication, and hopes and dreams were gone. It came down to survival. We hated what was happening to us, but couldn't stop the process.

I hated my husband and the fact that he was dealing coke. He had to deal to support our habits. I hated the people who would call or come to our house. I hated waking up at 3:00 A.M., looking for him, and finding he wasn't home. He would be out scoring drugs or selling them. I hated everything about my life, especially HIM. I used to wish he was cheating on me with another woman, because I could compete with another woman. I just couldn't compete with cocaine. It got to the point where most normal wives would get a divorce. My solution was to have him murdered. That way I could collect the insurance money. I knew the people to ask to do the job. The only problem was that my husband was their connection. They wouldn't want to kill their dealer, especially since he was a dealer who would front them, or anyone, anything they wanted.

We were the world's most unsuccessful dealers. No one ever sold more and made less than we did. We would always say, "Okay, this time we'll buy the coke, cut it, sell it, and have all the rest for ourselves for free." It always sounded so good, but it just never happened. Just like all the plans and dreams that we talked about during our famous "lude raps" never happened. Life itself with cocaine can never really happen. So, at the end of our using, I did finally tell my husband to get out.

When my wife told me I had to leave, it was the most devastating blow of my life. I never thought I would ever lose my wife and family. But here I was, desperate and afraid. I told her I would go to a meeting. I thought that a meeting would save my marriage. So I went and sat in the meeting, a broken man with no hope, thinking only about how I was going to get my next hit. Even though I didn't expect to, I heard a message from the people that shared. They, too, had lost all hope and all the good in their lives. Now that they were in the Program, and didn't use drugs or drink anymore, their lives had gotten better. I left that meeting with something I didn't have when I went in: HOPE.

I came running home from the meeting, "high" with the

hope that maybe it could happen for us as well. When I walked in the door my wife looked into my eyes and said, "Okay, what drugs have you taken? I want some." I said, "No, you don't understand. This meeting I went to was unbelievable. These people have gone through what we're going through, come out on the other side of this horrible existence, and are living happy, productive lives." I wanted her to come to see what I was talking about and, perhaps, find the hope that I had discovered. So we went to our first meeting together.

I was clean and sober, but my wife wasn't. She did her normal "just to function socially" routine, before going out: smoke a joint, drop a lude, and snort some coke — what she thought was the perfect high for a meeting.

I didn't know what to wear for a meeting, so I chose an old raincoat. When I got to the meeting I was sure I didn't belong. The one thing that I do remember was that the speaker said she looked in the mirror and hated the person she saw looking back. She said she saw a dirty little broad. I identified with that feeling, because that was exactly how I felt. I sat and cried for the rest of the meeting.

It took four days, a series of God-shots, and a lot of loving and caring people for me to finally surrender to the fact that I, too, was an addict and alcoholic. I regret that it took me those four days because now my husband has four days more sobriety than I, and he never lets me forget it. When his C.A. birthday rolls around, at 12:01 A.M., he wakes me up and says to me, "How many years do you have?" For four long days I have to listen to this, because for those four days, if he has seven years, I have six, and so on. But I always tell him "it's quality sobriety, not quantity that counts."

So we started our sober journey together and continued to go to meetings every day. We were two crazy newcomers, living together without a clue. This was the first time in our lives together that we were ever totally sober. All of a sudden, all the things we did loaded, we had to do sober. We didn't know you could go to a party, the movies, or make love sober.

These all seemed like impossibilities. One day, after about two weeks of sobriety, we looked at each other and she said, "You mean we're never going to smoke a joint again for the rest of our lives?" I said, "No way. Let's forget this Program thing!" Then my wife said one of the two things that has helped us the most: "Well, they say this works one day at a time. Maybe we could do that." I agreed. So we continued on and got very involved in the Program. We got sponsors, and we started working the Steps.

They told us to be of service, so we helped at meetings with coffee, setting up, and greeting people. Basically anything that was suggested, we did; especially working with others. When we were new, we worked with others that were newer. If we had ten days, we could help someone with five days, and tell them how we stayed sober for ten days.

We addicts can help other addicts like no one else can. The newcomers believe us. They know we have been through the same hell as they have, because we know exactly how they feel. Only addicts know what it's like to run out of drugs when you don't want to be out. Only another addict knows that horrible feeling of desperation, loneliness, and remorse. So we came to find out that our terrible experience with cocaine was going to be our greatest asset. By sharing this experience with others, we not only help them, but we also help ourselves to recover. We learned we must give this Program away in order to keep it. Anytime newcomers, especially couples, came into the Program, they were brought to us and were told that we got sober together. Those who brought the newcomers to us would then say, "Tell them how you did it." So, working with others became a big part of our program.

Things seemed to be improving for us. Slowly but surely, our lives were getting better. Still, there was something wrong. I was really happy and loving at the meetings. I was working with newcomers. I was kind to them. I was loving and giving to these strangers like they were my family. I would then go home to my family and yell and scream for the slightest reason. I was treating strangers with more love and respect than my wife and daughter. One night, at home after a meeting, my wife said something and I started screaming at her. Finally, she threw up her hands and screamed out, "Wait a minute, who do you think you're yelling at? I'm an addict and an alcoholic." I just shut up immediately. I was stunned. I had never thought of my wife as a fellow addict. So we were faced with a great problem that we had to find a solution to. I said to her, "What should we do?" She replied with the second thing that helped us: "Why don't we treat each other like newcomers? Why don't we give each other the same love, respect, tolerance, kindness, and understanding we give to newcomers?"

Well, that's been our motto and our guide to rebuilding a new and loving life together. Through the Program, we have both found a loving God of our own. He has blessed us with the gift of sobriety and another chance at life together.

By working and living the Steps of the Program on a daily basis, all of the love that was lost has come back, even stronger than before. The respect that was gone has returned. The trust that was severed has been repaired. The communication lines that were down are up again. But most of all, the Program has given us both our dignity and a sense of self-worth. I am a success today because I am a good husband and father and my wife's best friend, not because of what I do for a living. All of my self-esteem was wrapped up in my job. I am no longer what I do for a living. I am somebody. I feel good about me because I am worthy and deserve good things.

I have become the woman I have always wanted to be. I like the person I see in the mirror. I am no longer a victim. In fact, I am a functioning, successful woman who cares about other people's needs, not just my own needs. I am proud of what I have become. I have learned through the Program how to be a loving wife, mother, and, most of all, friend.

They say that this Program is an inside job with great rewards for those who work it. The good news is that anyone who wants it can have it. Anyone who has a dream can see it come true in sobriety. All you have to do is identify the dream, and this Program of action will help you achieve and surpass it. Sometimes, the greatest dreams are very simple. For us, just waking up in the morning and feeling okay was a dream come true. To be able to get through a day feeling at peace, even with unresolved problems going on in our lives, was a miracle.

This Program has given us a new way of life and a design for living we never thought possible. We have learned that we must look at the "big picture" and not focus on the little things that are wrong. If 98% of our lives is good, we no longer have to focus on the bad 2%, but rather on the good 98%. We know that whatever problems we have today will be resolved, as long as we stay in the solution and not in the problem.

We realize now that we each have a measure of self-worth, and that it's okay to be successful and for good things to happen. We see that we had just as hard a time accepting success as we did failure. So we now use the Serenity Prayer to help us through the good times and say, "God, grant us the serenity to accept the things we cannot change." We can't change the fact that life is good today. So, if we like what we're getting, we keep doing what we're doing. If we don't like what we are getting, we have to change what we are doing.

We wish everyone may find what we have found. It's here, not hidden. You just have to go for it. We realize that we may not be exactly what we want to be, and not precisely what we could be, but thank God we are not what we used to be.

24

SAVE A PRAYER

This atheist's mind suddenly cleared, and he knew that he had found a God he could understand.

*T*HE PORTION OF the Big Book entitled "How It Works" states: "If you have decided you want what we have and are willing to go to any length to get it — then you are ready to take certain steps." This addict has come to believe that the "it" referred to is a spiritual awakening. After my spiritual experience, I made the decision that I wanted to live by spiritual principles. I got into action by taking stock of myself, confessing my character defects, making restitution to those to whom I was able, and continuing to do so while I listened for the answers to my prayers.

On a quest to improve myself, I commit a portion of each day to physical fitness, running, bicycling, and baseball. I also seek to find happiness in simple things, as a child would. I try not to let the world get to me. I can do this by reliving the things I enjoyed as a kid: watching movies, building a toy airplane, or skipping rocks across the pond. I also pay close attention to what I eat to help maintain a healthy body.

My spiritual life is centered around a loving, forgiving, merciful God to whom I willingly give all my love and conscious thought. I am His servant. I believe and have been shown that He will care for and provide for me.

Each day I try to keep my thoughts positive and search out the good that is in all people and all situations, because I believe that my perceptions of myself and my attitude toward others affect how I am perceived in the world. I also believe that success begins with a dream and becomes reality through faith.

My life started out well enough. My parents had no addictions, didn't drink, and practiced spiritual principles.

They gave me love and guidance and nurtured me. They taught me about reality.

My good upbringing, however, did not prepare me for school. The other children were cruel to me and jealous of me because I was a happy and gifted child.

My dream was to become an astronaut. Therefore, I strove to excel at sports, science, and mathematics, which were taught to me by my father; as well as music and art, which were taught to me by my mother.

In high school my self-will went into action. I could no longer be tolerant and forgiving. Contrary to my parents' teachings, I had let resentments build up. I joined my peers and began drinking. With my alcohol abuse, my grades began to drop and so did my performance in sports. I no longer regarded my parents as loving and nurturing, but I had new friends, plus a girlfriend to take to the prom! My dreams of becoming an astronaut faded away; I went to art school instead.

I didn't fit in at the art school because I took science and mathematics courses as electives. In an attempt to fit in, I began taking drugs. In my senior year, I went on a mystical quest. Bored with art school, I studied philosophy and religion so that I could find God. My parents had taught me that God loved me, yet Sunday school taught me that God would unmercifully punish me. I wanted to find a God for myself. On this path, I read about a man who became enlightened by eating peyote. This seemed simpler than prayer, meditation, and logical philosophical practices. Tempted by the easy way, I ate a peyote button. I thought I saw God and that I was enlightened — everyone else thought I was just crazy.

Before I could be admitted to an asylum, my parents intervened and brought me home to love and nurture me back to reality. When I realized what had happened, I was so ashamed that I would not leave my parents' house; I would sit up in my attic bedroom and play guitar, looking out on the world from the window.

To get me out of the house, my sister gave me a puppy. Part of the responsibility of taking care of the puppy was taking him outdoors. On one of those excursions, I met a high school boy who became my only friend. He won my trust and would visit me in the attic. He encouraged me to begin playing my guitar in a band. Soon I was performing gigs on the road. The night of my last gig it rained terribly. My van was almost washed off the road. The next day I sensed that something was wrong. When I phoned home, I found out that my friend's car had washed off the road and that he was in a coma.

That night I drank with a purpose: to not feel anything. The next morning on the way home, as I watched the sun rise, I knew that my friend had died. A strange peace and happiness came over me, as though he was with me, telling me that he was joyful.

After the funeral, I became angry with God. I blamed Him for all that had happened to me. I was angry that He had let me get into trouble at school. I was angry that He had taken my friend from me. I was angry that there were cutbacks in the space program while I was in high school. Then the thought came to me that if there was no God, I couldn't be punished on Judgment Day. To die and find nothing seemed a more comforting thought than fire and brimstone. So I became an atheist and set about gathering proof of the nonexistence of God. As each day passed, my anger and bitterness grew.

I was introduced to cocaine by a girlfriend in my band. She got me to quit the band, cut my hair, start engineering school, and get a job. It was what she wanted me to do. I, in turn, wanted her to quit using cocaine because she loved cocaine more than she loved me. She left me on the spot. I then took a job in sales and traveled extensively. It was lonely on the road, so I spent my evenings in bars, looking for people to score for me, and feeding my addiction.

My bitterness towards God continued to grow. I twisted my scientific knowledge to support the nonexistence of God. In mathematics, a pure science, I saw evidence of a Higher Order, but I refused to believe, and vigorously denied, the possibility of a God.

My cocaine use escalated. I began smoking cocaine with my sister and her boyfriends who dealt. Eventually, my sister started attending a Twelve Step program and quit using cocaine. I wanted to quit also, but when I saw the word "God" in the Third Step, I balked. I denied that I really had a problem, and began using even more.

Later, I agreed to attend a meeting, even though I was really high and drunk at the time. I felt uneasy as people, who I was sure were aware that I was high, approached me. They looked at me with love and asked me to keep coming back. I was jonesing out of control and said nothing.

I had my sister take me to my weekend home — Mom's house; during the week I was homeless. When I found that Mom wasn't home, I went to the attic, filled my pipe and, in an attempt to forget about the people I had just met, took the biggest hit I could pull. My ears instantly went into long-metal-tunnel mode as I shut off the torch and dropped the pipe. Then my body began to convulse. My heart raced and then stopped. I couldn't move my arms to remove the pipe that was burning my leg. Then I lost my sight, as if someone had pulled the cable off the television antennae terminal. I felt alone, cold, and afraid. It was then that I prayed to God, "Please don't let me die like this. I deserve to die and I have no right praying, but I just don't want my mother to find me here tomorrow with this pipe next to me. Please, for my mother's sake."

Somehow, I lived that night and my mother did not have to suffer the humiliation of her son dying a cocaine addict's death. While sitting at home recovering from that incident,

I looked at a picture of my deceased father and had the feeling that he could still see me. I made a decision then not to smoke or use cocaine anymore. However, I felt that I could quit without going to meetings. I thought all I needed was will-power and some good physical exercise.

The next day was a classic warm New England day, possibly the last of the season, and a perfect one for a bicycle ride. I pulled my racer down and headed out. I had put in quite a ride and decided that the perfect finish would be a trip to the top of the hills near my home. It was quite a struggle, but cresting the hill and accelerating downwards made it all worthwhile. Then, as I hit top speed, my front tire exploded. I met the pavement violently, my head impacting with a hollow sound that reminded me of a coconut being split.

Paramedics, police, and family were soon on the scene. I thought that they were all overreacting to my accident, but when I saw the expression on my mother's face, I knew that the pain in my head was serious. I recalled the prayer of several days before: that I didn't want my mother to see me die of an overdose. I realized that perhaps my prayer was being answered.

I understood what it meant to be powerless over everything. I realized that I really was powerless; that whether I was to live or die was not within my control. At that moment, I wanted to live more than I ever had in my whole life. Then, an out-of-body experience began. Looking down upon the scene, I reflected on my life; how all the things I had ever wanted no longer meant anything at all. I reflected on what a happy and trouble-free day this had been. A peace came over me and I gazed at the sunset one last time. I said the second prayer of my life, "Thank you for today. I didn't deserve to have had a day like this." I then found quiet acceptance in waiting.

I awoke in the hospital where I had to spend a few days under observation. Several weeks after my accident, my sister relapsed. When she finally came home I stayed up all night to talk to her, reassure her, and keep her from going out. Well into the night, I began to tell her about the disease of cocaine addiction and how it would use resentments, fears, guilt, and anger to keep us under its control. My sister had a strange look on her face. She was puzzled that I knew of a program that I was not a part of. I explained that a voice which came from within was providing me with this new understanding. I explained what I had experienced the day of the accident: that when I finished my prayer and looked upon the world for the final time, it began to glow with an incredible light that became brighter than anything and filled everything, until it was all that I could see. It had filled me with love, comfort, and warmth. I felt forgiven, loved, and accepted. My sister said that most people would call that God. My mind suddenly cleared, and I knew that I now had a God whom I understood.

That inner voice stayed with me as I recovered from my accident. Each day it would ask, "Wouldn't you like to go to a meeting?" And I did go to C.A. meetings. In the meetings I found people who accepted me and loved me. In the rooms of Cocaine Anonymous I've found all my new friends.

One night, while I was helping another man clean coffee-pots at a meeting, he asked me why I didn't participate in the open prayer conducted at the end of the meeting. I replied that I believed in religious freedom, and, though I respected and tolerated his right to pray to God, I had my own God that I followed.

The man asked, "Are you a Buddhist? A Hindu? A Muslim?" I replied that I wasn't anything. Then he asked me what my God told me to do. For this I had no prepared answer. At a loss, I remembered that my parents had taught me to bow my head, silence my thoughts, and listen to the voice that comes from a place between my heart and stomach and speaks to me through feelings of understanding. So I did this and asked, "What do you want me to do?" The voice replied that I should love the little voice inside me before all else and that I must stay pure in heart, mind, and body so that I could hear Him. When I told this to the man, he asked, "Is that it?" So I went back to that place and asked "Is there anything else?" The voice said only one more thing — that I must go out and love others as much as I possibly could. When I told this to the man, he exclaimed that his God told him to do the same thing! He then asked me whether I had a name for my God.

I thought of my favorite movie which ends with an Inuit Indian prayer: "I think over again my life's small adventures, my fears — those small ones that seemed so big, and for all the vital things I had to get and reach. But there was only one Great Thing, the only thing: to live to see the Great Day that dawns and the Light that fills the world." Recalling my vision after the accident, I told him that I called my God "the Light that fills the world."

He said that his God was called "the Light of the world." Suddenly I realized that his God was the same as my God. I understood the meaning of the two simple words: our Father. I saw that deep down, I was the same as my friend, no better and no worse. So I came to understand that anonymity, the loss of self, was the spiritual foundation of all things.

I was a cocaine addict and an atheist and yet God did not have me suffer the slow, miserable death I was headed for. Instead, he let me live for another day and brought me to the rooms of Cocaine Anonymous where people love me, teach me how to love others, and welcome me.

Today, I awaken to see the dawn of another day. I know that God loves me and wants good things for me. In my heart, I save a prayer that I wish for everyone and say to many people, "Vaya con Dios — may you go with God."

25

LIVING FOR THE MOMENT
This woman has found that when she keeps the faith, she can't have the fear, and that what happens tomorrow is none of her business.

LL MY LIFE I felt like I didn't belong. I was raised in a very dysfunctional family. My mother and father separated while my mom was still pregnant with me. She was a practicing alcoholic until I was fifteen. My mother raised my brother and me alone and I never knew what it was like to have a father around.

As a child, I was very sensitive. I blamed myself for the absence of my parents. I thought that somehow it was my fault that my father never came to visit me. I couldn't understand why he didn't want to be a part of my life, and I felt that I just wasn't good enough. I also blamed myself for my mother's drinking. I thought that if I could just somehow do the right things, she could be happy. I had no self-worth by the time I was twelve and felt like a bad and worthless person.

I tried really hard to fix my mom because I thought it was my fault and my responsibility. I fought, cried, and pleaded with her and even poured her liquor down the drain. I thought that if I could just get her to stop drinking, my life would be okay. My brother reacted completely differently than I did: he just went into his room, shut the door, and pretended nothing was happening. We never discussed her drinking problem, and I thought that all families were like ours. I didn't realize that what was going on was not healthy.

By this time, I was very suicidal and just wanted the pain to go away. I then discovered marijuana. I loved the high, and suddenly I could bear the pain I was feeling inside. I began getting high on a daily basis and would sometimes leave home for three days at a time. This was fine with my mother, because then she could drink all she wanted, and no one would bother her.

When I was fourteen, I used cocaine for the first time. The euphoria was wonderful. I could now face the reality of my life as long as I stayed loaded. My brother was selling cocaine out of his bedroom, and I always managed to find his stash. It didn't matter to me that I was stealing; I just needed to be high. I couldn't avoid coming down and, when I did, I was left with myself and all the empty, worthless feelings.

When I was fifteen, I took an overdose of pills and ended up in a psychiatric hospital. At first I was angry, but soon decided I liked it there because it was a vacation from my life at home. I went back three times in that same year. Some of the kids at school thought I was crazy, but I didn't care. All I wanted was to be high or to die.

During all of this, my mother got sober and went to a Twelve Step fellowship. This was my first exposure to the Program. I saw her life change and get progressively better. I heard about the Principles and watched her work them in her life. I knew that this Program worked, and I was grateful for my mother's sobriety, but had no interest in sobriety for myself. I didn't feel powerless yet and, besides, I wasn't a drinker like her.

When I was nineteen, I smoked crack for the first time. It made me feel like I had never felt before, and I obsessed immediately. All I could think of was the next hit. About this time, I got into a really sick relationship that lasted four years. I chose someone who was worse off than I was, so I could focus on him and not deal with myself. Once again, I had someone in my life to try to fix. I guess that's not too surprising, considering "enabler" was the only role I ever learned to play.

I used to try to straighten out and keep away from the drugs on my own because I wanted to prove to myself that I wasn't powerless. I would stop for months at a time and, therefore, justify my next binge. My boyfriend would stay out all night and get loaded. I would get jealous and angry because he was getting high and I wasn't. I finally told him that if he wanted to stay with me, he had to go to Cocaine Anonymous and get sober; this was the first time I got involved with C.A. The thing that really struck me was all the love in those rooms. For the first time, I had a sense of belonging. I finally felt that I was a part of, and that I had true friends. Even so, I was there for the wrong reasons. I wasn't there for myself yet. Consequently, after several months, I left the Program and went back to my old way of life.

Shortly thereafter, my boyfriend received a $40,000 inheritance. This is what it took to make me hit bottom. Within six weeks, we were broke and homeless. My life had become complete insanity. I had lost my job, my home, my credit, 40 pounds, and what little self-worth I had left. It had all happened so fast, I couldn't believe it. It was like it all happened in a fog, and one day everything was gone. I didn't care about my life anymore. All that mattered to me was staying high so that I didn't have to face my reality. Sometimes I tried to smoke myself to death, but God had other plans for me. I lived on the streets and in my car for six months. My friends were prostitutes and street people. My boyfriend started to beat me violently. I went to jail three times. When my boyfriend started sleeping with a prostitute, I put up with it because I felt he was all I had left, and I didn't want to be out there alone. The three of us even lived together in my car for awhile. It got really sick.

One day, my boyfriend took off with his prostitute and left me behind. I had nothing now; I didn't even have shoes on my feet. I was sober for the first time in months, and the reality of what had become of my life hit me like a ton of bricks. I began sobbing uncontrollably; I cried for a good two hours. I decided to go sell myself on the street because I hated myself so much and wanted to punish myself. At the very moment that I had that thought, I heard a man's voice. He said, "I know you're hurting right now and you don't want to talk, but I just wanted to leave something with you." Then he put a Bible in my hands. I never looked up and saw this man's face, but I believe that he was an angel sent by my Higher Power. I am not a religious person, but I am very spiritual. At that moment, I had hope. I felt God was telling me, "I'm here with you. You're not alone." I knew I didn't have to punish myself and that somehow things would be okay. I didn't get sober then, but I believe that was a spiritual awakening for me. Afterwards, I knew I never had to be alone again.

Not long after, I was back with my boyfriend, living in the desert. I had reached a point at which I was so sick of this relationship that it felt like a ball and chain. I wanted more out of life and I knew that I had choices. I ended the relationship, moved back in with my mother, and got sober.

I called a friend in the Program and asked him to take me to a meeting. I got involved in C.A. again, and most of the friends I had met there before were still sober. They were all there for me and, once again, I felt a part of. I got a job. I started working the Steps. My life was coming together again. I took commitments and became willing to do things that scared me because I wanted to stay sober and to grow.

In my second month of sobriety, I decided to get tested for the HIV antibody because I knew my boyfriend had been with that prostitute. The test came back positive. I never believed that something like this could really happen in my life, but it did. I felt like my worst nightmares had come true. I felt like God had abandoned me and I couldn't understand why He was doing this to me now, when I was trying so hard to turn my life around. I went through a lot of anger. It took me a long time to accept it. But the miracle of it all is that I didn't drink or use. I just kept going to those meetings. I felt really alone for a long time. Nobody really knew what to say to me or how to handle the situation. At times, I felt like I was losing my mind and I thought that if I had to feel one more thing, I might die from the pain. I didn't. I knew I had to go on, though. I just had to keep walking through the days, one day at a time.

When I decided to start sharing about it in meetings, I was really scared because I didn't want to be rejected. But God was telling me that this was what I was supposed to do. I just had this overpowering feeling in my gut, and I knew that I had to do it. This is what freed me. For myself, I had to carry the message of my story. I know today that I can offer some hope to the addict who is still suffering. That brings me a lot of comfort; it gives my past some purpose. I also know today that I don't have to drink or use no matter what. Facing such tragedy in early sobriety gave me a strong foundation. I can be an example, showing that this Program works.

Living for the moment is really important to me now. I know that the time to do all those things I planned on doing someday is today. That's what living is all about. This moment is the only reality I have. Whenever I get scared or anxious, I ask myself, "What's happening in this moment?" That usually calms me down. The reality right now is that there are a lot of people out there who are really suffering, and I have never had it better. I want to give all that I can in this life. I have been blessed with the opportunity to carry the message.

My life has gotten progressively better since I got sober. I could not put into words how much I have grown. When I first got sober, I was so full of fear that it was overwhelming. I felt like a twelve-year-old in a twenty-four-year-old woman's body. I didn't feel comfortable in an adult situation, and I thought for sure that everybody could see right through me. When "The Promises" were read at meetings, stating that fear of people will leave us, I thought that it would be a miracle if that ever happened to me. I still have fear, but it doesn't run my life anymore. By facing my fears, they have less and less power over me. I guess miracles do happen.

I am working full-time and going to school at night. I am working toward getting a degree, which is something I could never have accomplished when I was getting loaded. It's amazing what a difference sobriety makes. All I do is show up and do what's suggested by the teacher, and I'm successful. I know today that I can be or do anything I want to in life, as long as I'm willing to do the footwork. By working this Program and these Steps in my life, I have learned that I am unlimited; my Higher Power made me that way. All I need to do is get up each day and do what's in front of me. I have turned my life and my will over to God. When I keep the faith, I can't have the fear, and what happens tomorrow is none of my business.

My mother has been sober for eleven years now and we not only have a relationship, but also a friendship. My father and I talk on a regular basis. I've learned to let go of my expectations and accept him as he is. I am in a happy, loving relationship and plan to be married in a few months. That is something that I thought would never happen in my life. These are all gifts of sobriety.

I work Steps One, Two, and Three on a daily basis and I not only apply them to my disease of addiction but also to my disease of HIV. Life has taken on a whole different perspective for me now. I am so grateful for each day and all the love I have in my life. I thank God all the time because I have happiness today and my life has so much meaning. I feel that I have so much to give now, and I'm so grateful that I didn't have to die out there on the street. Thanks to my Higher Power and Cocaine Anonymous, if I die tomorrow, my life will have a happy ending.

26

LEAVING LINES BEHIND
She thought everything seemed fine...until it wasn't.

*W*RITING MY STORY isn't too different from chairing a meeting: I don't know in advance what's going to be said. I've asked my Higher Power to guide me. That is a big change from what I first told my sponsor about a Higher Power, but then, everything is different than it was before recovery.

I used cocaine for seventeen years. Looking back, it's impossible to calculate how much I gave up and chose not to participate in so that I might use cocaine instead. Today I believe the loss to be the living experiences that passed me by. I spent so many years in dark bars and houses.

I am an only child of parents who were close to 50 when I was born. I was wanted and have no early horror story. I remember my earliest years as being safe and happy. My father died when I was ten, after a year's battle with cancer. While he was sick, no one talked about it. I only knew what was wrong by overhearing the adults whisper their secrets. At some age, we all experience the loss of a parent and it affects us forever. I thought I was an adult because my father had died, and believed my childhood was over. When we returned from the funeral, I boxed up all my toys and put them in the garage. Thirty years have passed since his death, and I still miss him. The pain of that loss is still not healed.

Just a few years later, I found LSD and all the other drugs of the sixties. I loved them all. They were the foundation of all of my actions, activities, and beliefs. In junior college, a teacher turned me onto my first cocaine experience. I didn't become a daily user right away; that took a few years, but I had found my drug of choice. What I did not find were goals of any sort. I had no major, no aspirations, and no dreams. I had a way of life, a drug user's way of life. After four years at a two-year college, I quit and took a job as a waitress.

Drugs and alcohol were everywhere. I had dealt some before, but dealing cocaine in the mid-seventies was a real moneymaker. I only quit dealing after a gun was put into my ear by a "friend." It was early enough in my disease that I could make the choice to stop dealing, but I was unable to stop using. That friend with a gun died a few years ago, alone in a filthy alley. I heard people who had kissed up to him when he had all the drugs cheer his demise. His wife of many years had left him. She, too, died of heart failure while snorting a celebratory line on Thanksgiving Day — there are no old practicing addicts.

I changed jobs, homes, and friends often in the next years. I met a man who used drugs like I did, and we married in a blackout. We were two sick addicts who knew nothing of intimacy. Our marriage was a war zone and my role was to be the victim.

We didn't make it much past a year. During this insanity, I was also a workaholic. I moved into management and then into corporate accounting. My relationships were with the people I worked with; needless to say they used and drank the way I did. I began to deal again, believing it would be different this time. I went from making a lot of money, to breaking even, to losing money at every turn, in just a couple of years.

The last few years of my using are vague. My coping skills were gone. My phone was for outgoing calls only. I was unable to answer the ring of the unknown caller. I could not open my mail, clean my house, or be a friend. I neglected my elderly mother, forgot my oldest friends, and found that my only voice was a sarcastic one. I was always trying to change or enhance what I was feeling. My world was getting smaller, and the terror was getting bigger. I began to see how hopelessly hooked I was. I could do nothing without cocaine. I was many thousands of dollars in debt and losing ground. I was arrested for using stolen credit cards, but amazingly was never arrested for drugs or drunk driving. I deserved both many times over. I had no emotions; I had become an uninterested observer of my life.

Somehow I found out about Cocaine Anonymous meetings. I attended every night for several weeks. When I had to go out of town, my disease went with me. It told me I had overreacted, that I could still have a cocktail. By the time the second drink was ordered, I was on the phone arranging a deal. Alcohol and cocaine are inseparable for me. I know I cannot drink without being taken back into the insanity of using.

The next eight months of "incomprehensible demoralization" were the worst, and the most desperate, of my using career. I had no idea how to change the course I was on. Once I found myself at home with my hand on the front door knob, not knowing if I had just come home or if I was going out. That was the moment I knew I couldn't go on the same way. I called a number I'd gotten eight months before, and within 24 hours I was in a 28-day recovery program.

When I went into the program, I told no one I was there. On the first family day, when everyone was having visitors, I had no one and was feeling lonely and sorry for myself. Those were the feelings I was most afraid of. I was filled with a gut-wrenching, gotta-have-it urge to get high. This was the first time I had that feeling but did not use. It was the last time I felt the need to use as strong as it was that day. I went to my room and asked a Power greater than myself, who I did not believe in, to help me. I don't remember what distraction occurred, but looking back, something happened and I got through that time. I have had the thought of using since that time, but never the absolute compulsion I experienced that afternoon in the recovery hospital.

I heard a lot about being willing, and I knew I could do that. I went to a lot of meetings. I talked to my sponsor about all the new experiences and the miracles. I learned about her Higher Power, as I slowly accepted one of my own. The Program taught me how to show up for life. No matter what, I went to meetings and did not use mind-altering substances. My sponsor became my roommate for a year. She introduced me to many different people and helped me maintain an open mind. She taught me that my recovery is a process, not an event. The process changes, and is painful at times, but it is a healthy path.

My spiritual, emotional, and physical health have all improved dramatically. When I was two years clean and sober, I got my chip with my ex-husband, who got his seven-year chip. We made amends, and I let go of the years of hate and resentment. I saw the miracle of recovery in his life and in my own.

On my next birthday I will pick up a six-year chip. I have fallen in love in this Program. I have an appreciation for my life I never had before. There are moments when I am delighted to be me. Some wonderful women have honored me by working the Steps with me and letting me see their lives change.

I had never been interested in group activities, yet in recovery I have participated in many activities and in different types of service. I share a feeling of belonging with the people in this Fellowship. There are some people who are seen only at annual events, some much more frequently; but we are all people who have accepted the gift of recovery. We in Cocaine Anonymous are a group of people who are grateful to enjoy our lives — one day at a time.

APPENDICES

APPENDICES

A

SELF-TEST FOR COCAINE ADDICTION

1. Have you ever used more cocaine than you planned?

2. Has the use of cocaine interfered with your job?

3. Is your cocaine use causing conflict with your spouse or family?

4. Do you feel depressed, guilty, or remorseful after you use cocaine?

5. Do you use whatever cocaine you have almost continually until the supply is exhausted?

6. Have you ever experienced sinus problems or nosebleeds due to cocaine use?

7. Do you ever wish you had never taken that first line, hit, or injection of cocaine?

8. Have you experienced chest pains or rapid or irregular heartbeats when using cocaine?

9. Do you have an obsession to get cocaine when you do not have it?

10. Are you experiencing financial difficulties due to your cocaine use?

11. Do you experience an anticipation high just knowing you are about to use cocaine?

12. After using cocaine, do you have difficulty sleeping without taking a drink or other drug?

13. Are you absorbed with the thought of getting loaded even while interacting with a friend or loved one?

14. Have you begun to use drugs or drink alone?

15. Do you ever have feelings that people are talking about you or watching you?

16. Do you have to use larger amounts of drugs or alcohol to get the same high you once experienced?

17. Have you tried to quit or cut down on your cocaine use only to find that you could not?

18. Have any of your friends or family suggested that you may have a problem?

19. Have you ever lied to, or misled, those around you about how much or how often you use?

20. Do you use drugs in your car, at work, in the bathroom, in airplanes, or in other public places?

21. Are you afraid that if you stop using cocaine or alcohol, your work will suffer or you will lose your energy?

22. Do you spend time with people or in places you otherwise would not be around but for the availability of drugs?

23. Have you ever stolen drugs or money from friends or family?

If you have answered "yes" to any of these questions, you may have a cocaine problem. There is an answer — come to meetings of Cocaine Anonymous, read the literature, and join us — we want to help.

B

A HIGHER POWER

*A*S A NEWCOMER, you may have thought or said, "What's this talk about God? I came here to stop using cocaine, not to join a new religion." Don't feel alone. Many of us were put off with the talk about God when we first came to meetings.

It is easy enough to confuse the word spirituality with religion. As it relates to God, Cocaine Anonymous is a spiritual program, not a religious one. In C.A., we believe each individual can choose a Higher Power of his or her own. In short, a God of his or her own understanding.

If you are like many of us, you came to C.A. without a conscious belief in a Higher Power. Or, perhaps you chose to avoid a Higher Power because you were taught about a punishing God. It doesn't matter. All that is necessary to start is that you are open-minded to the idea that *some* Power greater than yourself may be able to restore you to sanity.

The first step in solving any problem is recognizing it. The same holds true in solving a problem with cocaine.

The second step in solving a problem is believing that there might be a solution. The fact that you've come to a C.A. meeting shows that you believe that there is a power of some kind, greater than yourself, that can help you get your life back in order. You have proven, just by showing up, that you believe that there must be some information, somewhere, you can use to get rid of your obsessions with cocaine, drugs, and/or alcohol. You have already started!

The third step in solving a problem, after having found evidence of a solution, is putting faith in that solution and trying it. That solution for us meant admitting that our management of the problem wasn't working. Cocaine Anonymous introduced us to a Power greater than ourselves that *could* manage our problem. That doesn't necessarily mean we have to turn our will and our lives over to the care of the God that we heard of in the past. It can mean trusting in a Power of our own understanding. This is the beginning of our Higher Power, God as we understand Him.

Some of us adopt, or come back to, a traditional God. Others see our Higher Power as some kind of force. Some define it as the force of the group, while others don't define it at all.

At first, it is sufficient for God, as you understand Him, to be the power that the group obviously has to help get rid of the obsession to use.

No one comes into Cocaine Anonymous to find God. We come to these rooms to get rid of a terrifying drug habit. Look around in a meeting. You are surrounded by people who came as a last resort. We came into these rooms emotionally, financially, and spiritually bankrupt. We have experienced all sorts of tragedies as a result of cocaine, drugs, and/or alcohol. We have lived many of the same horrors you have, yet today we are happy. We are free from the misery, terror, and pain of drug addiction.

As long as you are willing, your belief will grow. You will learn through your own experience and the experiences of others how a Higher Power can help you with your cocaine problem.

Maybe some of us were worse off than you; maybe some of us didn't hit as low a bottom as you. Still, the fact remains, that those of us who are recovering have come to believe that the power of the group or of a Higher Power of our own understanding can restore us to sanity.

After you are around the Program for a few weeks and months, you will begin to see changes in your thinking. You will begin to feel better. You will see changes in the other newcomers that came in with you. We call those changes miracles. If you are having trouble with the talk about God, remember:

- Be open-minded
- C.A. is a spiritual program, not a religious one
- All you have to do is to be willing to believe
- Your Higher Power can be the group as a whole
- You start with belief, your experience will come.

Don't leave before the miracle happens!

C

...AND ALL OTHER MIND-ALTERING SUBSTANCES

STEP ONE: We admitted we were powerless over cocaine and all other mind-altering substances — that our lives had become unmanageable.

*W*HAT EXACTLY DOES the "and all other mind-altering substances" part mean? I came to Cocaine Anonymous because *cocaine* had become a problem in my life.

We in Cocaine Anonymous, who have been around a while, hear this statement all the time from newcomers. If you read on, we will share with you how we learned that our real problem was not just cocaine or any specific drug; it was the disease of addiction.

Some of us never even used cocaine. There were other drugs that got us into trouble. Or, maybe it was the combination of cocaine, alcohol, marijuana, or heroin that had made our lives miserable. Cocaine Anonymous' First Step is viewed by our Fellowship as a "blanket" first step because all types of drug users are welcome as long as they have the desire to stop using.

In our using days, we rode drug roller coasters. There were drugs to come down with, drugs to go up with, and drugs to mellow out with. In recovery, we have discovered, sometimes the hard way, through relapse, that we could not control our use of any mind-altering substances. If our bodies were not absolutely drug-free, the compulsion to use was always lurking. We inevitably returned to our favorite drug, or went back to an old preference in chemicals. Whatever the drug, the problem of not being able to stop would resurface, usually stronger than before.

Here is an example: imagine that you have just run out of

cocaine and cannot get any more. What would you choose as it's substitute? Alcohol? Speed? Heroin? The list could go on and on. It really wouldn't matter what you'd substitute for cocaine. The point is that you would soon find yourself unable to stop using and would be worrying about when you would run out of your replacement drug.

ALCOHOL   Alcohol is a mind-altering chemical in liquid form. Many people don't realize that it is no different from cocaine, marijuana, painkillers, or tranquilizers in its ability to lead to addiction. One drink is never enough, just as one hit, fix, pill, or snort is never enough. We are masters at combining and substituting one drug for another to get high. Many of us never felt that alcohol was part of our problem. However, take away the drug of choice, substitute another, and eventually it becomes a problem drug.

PAINKILLERS   Our bodies and minds don't know the difference between drugs used for pain relief and drugs used for pleasure. It is wise to inform each of your physicians, from your dentist to your orthopedic surgeon, from your psychiatrist to your medical doctor, that you are a recovering addict. They might already know, especially if you have abused prescription drugs. Informing your doctors is suggested because they should keep this in mind before prescribing anything that could threaten your recovery.

Sometimes, the use of painkillers is necessary if you are suffering physically. Don't be alone with your worst enemy. We are people who like drugs — a lot! The drugs can talk to you and soon have you convinced that you need them more frequently than prescribed. Another recovering addict to talk to, an informed prescribing physician, and medication dispensed by someone other than yourself can all be helpful in preventing abuse.

TRANQUILIZERS, ANTIDEPRESSANTS, AND OTHER PRESCRIPTION DRUGS In sobriety we begin to experience feelings that had been buried deep within ourselves. Sometimes these feelings seem to surface all at once. Follow the advice of a physician who is aware that you are a recovering addict if it comes to the need to use tranquilizers, antidepressants, or other prescription drugs.

Abruptly stopping the use of such drugs can be dangerous and even deadly if not done under the guidance of an informed physician.

OVER-THE-COUNTER AND COMMONLY USED LEGAL DRUGS Over-the-counter and legal drugs, such as cough syrups that contain alcohol and/or codeine, diet pills that act like speed, and antihistamines that cause drowsiness and can be abused to induce sleep, can be just as addicting as street drugs. We suggest that you become a label reader. There are many more products on the market that contain mind-altering chemicals that can be dangerous to an addict who has the potential to abuse just about anything.

In summary, we suggest that you ask your doctor or pharmacist if you have questions that are unanswered. Be honest with your sponsor about what drugs you take or are prescribed to you. Uninformed addicts are a danger to themselves.

When you realize that you no longer need drugs to come down, go up, or maintain, you have experienced one of the many joys and freedoms of recovery. You have stopped using and have started to live.

D

CHOOSING YOUR SPONSOR

WHY SPONSORSHIP? By this time you may have gone to meetings and heard lots of talk about working the Steps, a power greater than ourselves and getting a sponsor. You may also have become aware that Cocaine Anonymous is based on the Twelve Steps of Recovery. But, if you're like many of us were, you're not sure what is meant by working the Steps, finding a Higher Power or getting a sponsor.

Many of us would not have been able to stay clean and sober were it not for the special one-to-one relationships with our sponsors.

C.A. may at first seem unfamiliar. During the early days of sobriety, it's a good idea to get a sponsor. At first, you might have a lot of questions and concerns, and a sponsor can devote more time to your individual questions than regular meetings allow. Sponsors can introduce you to other people at meetings. It might help you feel more comfortable at meetings to be with someone who knows his or her way around.

Although people at meetings respond to our questions willingly, that alone isn't enough. Many other questions occur to us between meetings; many of us find that we need constant, close support as we begin learning how to live sober.

WHAT IS A SPONSOR? A sponsor is a clean and sober addict who shares with you how they maintain their sobriety by working the Twelve Steps. The sponsor's primary tools are his or her experience, strength and hope.

There are no specific rules, but a sponsor should probably

be sober for a year or more and be enjoying his or her new life as a result of the Twelve Steps.

A sponsor was once a newcomer too, and has used the C.A. program to deal with problems similar to those the newcomer is now facing.

Sharing the lessons of what he or she has learned staying sober is what a sponsor is all about. On a one-to-one basis, a sponsor can share his or her experience, strength and hope in living a happy, joyous and free life.

Sponsors are not professional counselors and are not certified to offer legal, psychiatric or medical advice. Nor is a sponsor someone upon whom we can rely to get us jobs, clothing or food. Sponsors have been down the rocky road before and often can suggest where you can obtain the professional help you might need. Do not hesitate to call your sponsor. It may be hard at first to pick up the phone— we do not find it easy to ask for help. But remember, a sponsor has been there and knows how you feel.

FINDING A SPONSOR   Some of the ways we have gotten to know people and found a sponsor are:

- Listening to the feelings being shared at meetings.
- Asking members of the fellowship for their phone numbers, then actually calling and talking to them.
- Going to coffee after meetings with other sober addicts.
- Sharing at meetings.
- Asking others to recommend someone as a sponsor.

When choosing a sponsor, remember that this does not have to be a life-long relationship. Many of us have had different sponsors at different times in our sobriety. Others have had the same sponsor since early sobriety. The point is that YOU must take the initiative and reach out.

A DISCUSSION OF SPONSORSHIP   In C.A., experience has shown that it's best for men to sponsor men and women to sponsor women. This custom promotes quick understanding and reduces the likelihood of emotional distractions, which might take the newcomer's mind off the purpose of Cocaine Anonymous.

At times, we may feel uncomfortable with what our sponsor suggests. But remember sponsors have traveled the road before and are sharing their experience with us to help us through difficult times.

Which sponsor is best for you? No one but you can answer that question. Sponsors may share interests similar to yours, but may also be totally different. It's best to attend meetings and listen to what experienced individuals have to say about living the steps with strength and hope. Again, a sponsor only shares his or her experience, strength and hope. By sharing our difficulties with our sponsor on a one-to-one basis, it makes day-to-day living a lot easier and our struggle less lonely.

Remember, sponsors have lives outside C.A. They have families, jobs and other responsibilities. Although a sponsor will do whatever he or she can to help you maintain your sobriety, there will be times when a sponsor is truly unavailable. So what are we to do? Check listings for the next C.A. meeting, read the steps and literature, contact the local C.A. office, or pull out those telephone numbers of other recovering addicts and call. Keep an active telephone list of recovering addicts with you and above all CALL. Your call will be helping the other person as much as it helps you. Other recovering addicts know what you are experiencing and will sincerely help you through the rough times. But before you can get help, you have to reach out and ask for it. It's there, ready and willing to be shared.

A person may have more than one sponsor. Someone with two or more sponsors has a wider range of experience available to him or her. Others, however, feel that having only one sponsor promotes a more focused approach to the C.A. program.

It is never too late to get a sponsor. Whether you are a newcomer hesitant about "bothering" someone, or a member who has been around for some time trying to go it alone, sponsorship is yours for the asking. We urge you: DO NOT DELAY. We in C.A. want to share what we have learned with other addicts because experience has taught us that we keep what we have by giving it away.

Most members of Cocaine Anonymous owe their sobriety to the fact that someone else took a special interest in them and was willing to share a great gift with them. A C.A. member often finds that getting a good sponsor, talking frankly and listening can make the whole program open up as it never did before.

E

SUGGESTIONS FOR RELAPSE PREVENTION AND RECOVERY

RELAPSE — to fall back into a previous condition, especially after a partial recovery from illness.

As stated in our literature, we believe that our addiction is a disease; a disease from which we can recover, one day at a time. As with any other disease, the potential for relapse is very real and deadly. The greatest difference between our disease and say, that of cancer, is that we have a choice. It's with this fact in mind that we of Cocaine Anonymous wish to offer our experience as it relates to relapse — both prevention and recovery.

RELAPSE PREVENTION — the following suggestions have been found to be invaluable in the prevention of relapse by those of us in recovery in Cocaine Anonymous.

1) **Abstinence** We suggest that any person desiring recovery abstain from the use of any mind-altering substances. We have found that as addicts we possess an uncanny ability to switch drugs. Again, addiction is not the drug, it is the disease.

2) **Triggers** Many of us weren't aware of those things which prompted our using. We view these as triggers, some of which are as follows:

PLACES In recovery, we found it wise to be aware of our motives for being in certain places. Most of us found it necessary to stay away from clubs, parties, rock houses, pool halls, and other places where we used.

PEOPLE   It's difficult to understand, but necessary to do, and that's to stay away from our using friends. We had to be mindful that they too are sick and at no time are we stronger in our recovery than they are in their disease. They have the power to trigger our relapse both by and through their behavior.

DEALING   With this, many of us faced a dilemma. We were addicted to the money and the excitement. We dealt for power and for control. Many of us relapsed by dealing because we lost sight of our lack of personal power.

3) **Meetings**   We suggest at least one meeting a day for newcomers. We also suggest a meeting whenever you don't feel like you need one. We have found that when we *don't* want to go is when we *do* need to go. Again, meetings are where our collective experience, strength, and hope is shared.

4) **Keep in touch**   Keeping in touch with a sponsor or friend in recovery is an ideal way of keeping yourself focused on recovery.

5) **Hungry**   Don't get too hungry. While Cocaine Anonymous has no opinion on outside issues, we have found that it's difficult to maintain emotional balance without eating regularly throughout the day.

6) **Angry**   It is said that this emotion is best left up to those better equipped to deal with it. As people in recovery, we have found that lingering anger, whether justified or not, is better left to others. There is no shorter course to getting loaded than a run with anger and resentment.

7) **Lonely**   It's been our experience that an addict alone is in the worst possible company. Again, we suggest

meetings and fellowship. For those of us who isolated behind closet and bathroom doors or tinfoiled windows, being around others is at first an unnerving experience. After we tried it, and sincerely gave it some time, we found a new freedom and new friendships which we never dreamed possible.

8) **Tired**   It took some time for many of us to reach regular sleep habits. While we do not know of people dying of lack of sleep, we do know of many instances where a tired addict reached for that bump or jump start and relapsed.

9) **Action/work**   It's a rare case in which someone actually working the Steps has relapsed. We have found that as long as our focus is on the Steps and the action required to work them, relapse is a remote, rare thought.

10) **Phrases**   These simple sayings or prayers have helped many of us through difficult times:

THIS TOO SHALL PASS   It's difficult to remember, but in daily recovery, whatever the feeling or problem, it will pass.

SERENITY PRAYER   This prayer is not designed to make the problem disappear. Its purpose is to bring peace to the user.

FIRST THINGS FIRST   You can only do what's in front of you.

ONE DAY AT A TIME   Not for the rest of your life.

LET GO AND LET GOD   Do the footwork but leave the results up to your Higher Power.

11) **Signs of relapse**   The following are some of the
signs that have preceded relapses:

- I deny my fear
- I convince myself that "I'll never drink/use again"
- I decide that "not using" is all I need
- I try to force sobriety on others
- I become overconfident about my recovery
- I behave compulsively (overwork/underwork,
  overtalk/withdraw)
- I start isolating
- I make unrealistic or haphazard plans
- I live in the "there and then"
- I start daydreaming of failure
- I view my problems as unsolvable
- I avoid having fun
- I overanalyze myself
- I become irritated by friends/family
- I am easily angered
- I begin blaming people, places, things, and
  conditions for my problems
- I begin doubting my disease
- I eat irregularly (overeat/undereat, snack)
- I have these listless periods
- I sleep irregularly (oversleep/undersleep)
- I experience periods of deep depression
- I develop an "I don't care attitude"
- I hoard money, sex, or power
- I openly reject help
- I rationalize that drinking/using can't make my
  life worse than it is now
- I feel sorry for myself
- I have fantasies of social drinking/using
- I begin to lie consciously

- I increase my use of aspirin/non-prescription medications
- I am overwhelmed with loneliness, frustration, anger, and tension
- I begin visiting drinking/using "friends" and places
- I convince myself that I'm cured
- I lose control
- I tell myself that it's okay to deal — I can use the money; it'll be quick and easy.

WHAT IF YOU DO RELAPSE?

1) Call your sponsor, the hotline, or another sober member of Cocaine Anonymous. Stay in touch.

2) Keep going to meetings. The only requirement for membership is a *desire* to stop using.

3) Keep reaffirming your desire by getting newcomer chips.

4) Remember, no matter what...

Keep coming back! Allow us to love you until you can love yourself — it does work!

F

THE FIRST 30 DAYS

*W*ELCOME to Cocaine Anonymous. We are all here for the same reason — our inability to stop using cocaine. The first step towards solving any problem is understanding the problem.

THE PROBLEM   The problem, as we see it, consists of an obsession of the mind and a compulsion of the body. The obsession is a continued and irresistible thought of cocaine and the next high. Once we have given in to this thought, our bodies take over. Our compulsion consists of an absolute inability to stop using once we begin. Thus, our recovery begins with complete abstinence from cocaine and all other mind-altering substances. This allows us to begin living in the solution.

THE SOLUTION   We wish to assure you that there *is* a solution and that recovery *is* possible. It begins with abstinence and continues with practicing the Twelve Steps of recovery one day at a time.

Take it easy. Addiction is not a moral issue. Addiction is a disease — a disease that kills. Here are some suggestions to help you stay clean and sober for your first 30 days:

Abstinence   Do not use any mind-altering substances! Experience has shown us that the use of any mind-altering substance will ultimately lead us back to addiction in another form or to our drug of choice, cocaine.

A meeting a day   Attend at least one meeting a day or more. Meetings are where we go to share our experience, strength, and hope with each other.

Get a sponsor   It is a good idea to get a sponsor during your early days, when C.A. seems strange and new. A sponsor is simply a sober addict who can give you more time and attention than is available at meetings.

Use the telephone   Get phone numbers from C.A. members and use them. A vital part of our recovery process is reaching out to others. If no one is available, call Cocaine Anonymous.

One day at a time   We stay clean and sober one day at a time, and, when necessary, one hour or even one minute at a time; not one week, one month, or one year, just one day at a time.

As we get clean and sober, our feelings begin to surface. Cocaine helped us escape from ourselves; it altered our reality. It helped us cover up, avoid, and deaden our feelings. Getting clean and sober can be painful, but with help, we find our lives get better one day at a time.

When we attended our first C.A. meeting, we knew deep down inside that cocaine had become a problem in our lives. Seeing this was just the beginning. This is where the program of Cocaine Anonymous comes into play. We begin by surrendering and working the Twelve Steps of recovery.

Step One   *We admitted we were powerless over cocaine and all other mind-altering substances — that our lives had become unmanageable.*

Most of us disliked the idea of being powerless over anything. We thought that cocaine made us invincible and powerful, when, in actuality, it wiped us out financially, emotionally, physically, and spiritually. We were out of control and had reached the depths of despair. The extent to which our lives had become unmanageable, of course, was different for each of us. The fact remained that our lives had become unmanageable. Not until we got honest with ourselves and surrendered, did we begin to know peace.

Step Two *Came to believe that a power greater than ourselves could restore us to sanity.*

Step Two involves open-mindedness. Having admitted we were powerless over cocaine and all other mind-altering substances, we became open-minded enough to believe that a Power greater than ourselves could remove our obsession to use and restore us to sanity. This Power may be, but does not have to be, God. Many of us use the Fellowship of C.A. as our Higher Power. After all, what we had failed to do alone, we are succeeding in doing together.

Step Three *Made a decision to turn our will and our lives over to the care of God **as we understood Him.***

Cocaine Anonymous is a spiritual program, not a religious one. We claim spiritual progress rather than spiritual perfection. Some of us arrived with a God, while others used the group until they found a Higher Power of their own understanding. A key phrase in this Step is "*as we understood Him.*" In Cocaine Anonymous, each individual can choose a God of his own understanding.

As we worked the Twelve Steps of recovery, we began to see some of the Promises coming true in our lives:

If we are painstaking about this phase of our development, we will be amazed before we are halfway through. We are going to know a new freedom and a new happiness. We will not regret the past nor wish to shut the door on it. We will comprehend the word serenity and we will know peace. No matter how far down the scale we have gone, we will see how our experience can benefit others. That feeling of uselessness and self-pity will disappear. We will lose interest in selfish things and gain interest in our fellows. Self-seeking will slip away. Our whole attitude and outlook upon life will change. Fear of people and of economic insecurity will leave us. We will intuitively know how to handle situations which used to baffle us. We will suddenly realize that God is doing for us what we could not do for ourselves.

Are these extravagant promises? We think not. They are being fulfilled among us — sometimes quickly, sometimes slowly. They will always materialize if we work for them.[7]

---

[7]Reprinted from *Alcoholics Anonymous*, pages 83 & 84, with permission from A.A. World Services, Inc.

G

TOOLS OF RECOVERY

*T*HERE COMES A time when the cocaine stops working—a time when the coke, the other drugs, and all the madness become unbearable. By then, you just can't stop, so you manage to score and somehow survive and keep on using because, although it's killing you, cocaine has become the most important thing in your life. If, somehow, some way, you get a break from it, get free for a moment with a little clarity, you will know this may be your last chance. You must stop using now, and you are really scared. You want to stay away from cocaine, but you don't know how.

If you want to be clean and sober, you can be. If you want what we have, you can have it. No matter how much cocaine you have used or how low you have sunk, you can get away and stay away from cocaine. But you must do what we have done. Thousands of recovering cocaine addicts are living drug-free and own their lives again. They are doing this by actively using the tools of recovery in the program of Cocaine Anonymous. These are some of the tools that work for us:

TOTAL ABSTINENCE We who have lost control of our cocaine consumption must abstain from all mind-altering substances. Our experience is that our addiction is invariably triggered by the use of alcohol or other drugs. Just don't drink or use, no matter what.

MEETINGS This is where we meet other recovering addicts. What we failed to do alone we can do together. We share our experience, strength, and hope at meetings. We also learn valuable information about our disease and how the program of Cocaine Anonymous works in our lives. We suggest that you get a meeting directory and go to 90 meetings in 90 days.

LITERATURE   The books *Alcoholics Anonymous* (the "Big Book") and *Twelve Steps and Twelve Traditions* (the "Twelve and Twelve") of Alcoholics Anonymous are two of our most valuable tools of recovery. Cocaine Anonymous publishes numerous pieces of literature to further help the recovering addict.

SPONSOR   A sponsor is a recovering addict with more sobriety and Program experience than yourself who will help you work the Steps. He or she (same sex is recommended) should be someone you think you can communicate with. Begin looking for a sponsor immediately. You can change sponsors if the relationship doesn't work out.

THE TWELVE STEPS   Meetings may keep you sober for some time, but the Twelve Steps of Cocaine Anonymous are vital for a stable and happy recovery. The Steps of Cocaine Anonymous are the means by which we move from the problem of drug addiction to the solution of recovery. We learn about the Steps by reading the literature, by attending Step study meetings, and by working with a knowledgeable sponsor.

HIGHER POWER   We urge new members to explore whatever beliefs they may have in a Power greater than themselves. There are no religious requirements or beliefs necessary for membership. Some of us either lost our spirituality before we came to C.A. or have never had any spiritual beliefs. As we recovered, many of us experienced new or reawakened spiritual feelings. Be open-minded.

SERVICE   One of the keys to successful recovery is getting involved. Begin by getting and keeping commitments at meetings — make coffee; help clean up; put away chairs. Help yourself by helping others.

TELEPHONE   The telephone is our lifeline between meetings. Get phone numbers from other C.A. members.

We are usually shy about calling at first, but we must find a way to do it. We suggest you call someone in the Program daily.

ONE DAY AT A TIME   The thought of making a pledge to never use again can be discouraging. We stay clean and sober one day at a time, and, if necessary, one hour or even one minute at a time.

PRAYER AND MEDITATION   These are the tools with which we establish and improve our conscious contact with God, *as we understood Him*. We have found the Serenity Prayer to be very helpful:

God, grant me the serenity to accept the things I cannot change, courage to change the things I can, and wisdom to know the difference.

Make your recovery your number one priority. All your hopes and plans, your very survival, depend on a drug-free you. Staying away from cocaine and all other mind-altering substances may be the greatest challenge you will ever face. The early period can be tough. This does not mean you are not getting better. Beware of thoughts like "I don't feel good," or "This is not working." Recovery is a process and it takes time.

We hope that by using these tools you will find the same joy and freedom we have found. Just remember to be patient and keep coming back.

H

THE TWELVE STEPS OF COCAINE ANONYMOUS

We use the Twelve Steps of recovery because it has already been proven that the Twelve Step recovery program works.

1. We admitted we were powerless over cocaine and all other mind-altering substances — that our lives had become unmanageable.

2. Came to believe that a Power greater than ourselves could restore us to sanity.

3. Made a decision to turn our will and our lives over to the care of God *as we understood Him.*

4. Made a searching and fearless moral inventory of ourselves.

5. Admitted to God, to ourselves, and to another human being the exact nature of our wrongs.

6. Were entirely ready to have God remove all these defects of character.

7. Humbly asked Him to remove our shortcomings.

8. Made a list of all persons we had harmed, and became willing to make amends to them all.

9. Made direct amends to such people wherever possible, except when to do so would injure them or others.

10. Continued to take personal inventory and when we were wrong promptly admitted it.

11. Sought through prayer and meditation to improve our conscious contact with God *as we understood Him*, praying only for knowledge of His will for us and the power to carry that out.

12. Having had a spiritual awakening as the result of these steps, we tried to carry this message to addicts, and to practice these principles in all our affairs.

I

THE TWELVE TRADITIONS OF COCAINE ANONYMOUS

The Twelve Traditions are to the group what the Twelve Steps are to the individual.

1. Our common welfare should come first; personal recovery depends upon C.A. unity.

2. For our group purpose there is but one ultimate authority — a loving God as He may express Himself in our group conscience. Our leaders are but trusted servants; they do not govern.

3. The only requirement for C.A. membership is a desire to stop using cocaine and all other mind-altering substances.

4. Each group should be autonomous except in matters affecting other groups or C.A. as a whole.

5. Each group has but one primary purpose — to carry its message to the addict who still suffers.

6. A C.A. group ought never endorse, finance, or lend the C.A. name to any related facility or outside enterprise, lest problems of money, property, and prestige divert us from our primary purpose.

7. Every C.A. group ought to be fully self-supporting, declining outside contributions.

8. Cocaine Anonymous should remain forever nonprofessional, but our service centers may employ special workers.

9. C.A., as such, ought never be organized; but we may create service boards or committees directly responsible to those they serve.

10. Cocaine Anonymous has no opinion on outside issues; hence the C.A. name ought never be drawn into public controversy.

11. Our public relations policy is based on attraction rather than promotion; we need always maintain personal anonymity at the level of press, radio, television, and films.

12. Anonymity is the spiritual foundation of all our Traditions, ever reminding us to place principles before personalities.

Reprinted and adapted with the permission of A.A. World Services, Inc. The Twelve Traditions of Alcoholics Anonymous: 1. Our common welfare should come first; personal recovery depends upon A.A. unity. 2. For our group purpose there is but one ultimate authority — a loving God as He may express Himself in our group conscience. Our leaders are but trusted servants; they do not govern. 3. The only requirement for A.A. membership is a desire to stop drinking. 4. Each group should be autonomous except in matters affecting other groups or A.A. as a whole. 5. Each group has but one primary purpose — to carry its message to the alcoholic who still suffers. 6. An A.A. group ought never endorse, finance or lend the A.A. name to any related facility or outside enterprise, lest problems of money, property and prestige divert us from our primary purpose. 7. Every A.A. group ought to be fully self-supporting, declining outside contributions. 8. Alcoholics Anonymous should remain forever nonprofessional, but our service centers may employ special workers. 9. A.A., as such, ought never be organized; but we may create service boards or committees directly responsible to those they serve. 10. Alcoholics Anonymous has no opinion on outside issues; hence the A.A. name ought never be drawn into public controversy. 11. Our public relations policy is based on attraction rather than promotion; we need always maintain personal anonymity at the level of press, radio and films. 12. Anonymity is the spiritual foundation of all our Traditions, ever reminding us to place principles before personalities.

The Twelve Steps and Twelve Traditions are reprinted with permission of Alcoholics Anonymous World Services, Inc. Permission to reprint and adapt the Twelve Steps and Twelve Traditions does not mean that A.A. is affiliated with this program. A.A. is a program of recovery from alcoholism. Use of the Steps and Traditions in connection with programs and activities which are patterned after A.A., but which address other problems, does not imply otherwise.

C.A. PAMPHLETS

A Guide To The Twelve Steps
A Higher Power
...And All Other Mind-Altering Substances
A New High from H & I
Choosing Your Sponsor
Cocaine Anonymous InfoLine Numbers
Crack
Reaching Out to the Deaf and Hard of Hearing
Self-Test for Cocaine Addiction
Suggestions for Relapse Prevention and Recovery
The First 30 Days
The 7th Tradition (Where Does the Money Go?)
Tools of Recovery
To the Newcomer
What Is C.A.?
Tips on Staying Clean and Sober

Most of the above are available in Spanish and French

Order forms available from:
CAWSO, Inc.
P.O. Box 492000, Los Angeles, CA, 90049-8000

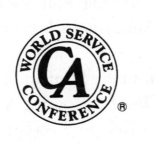